PARENT–TEEN THERAPY
FOR EXECUTIVE FUNCTION DEFICITS AND ADHD

Parent–Teen Therapy for Executive Function Deficits and ADHD

BUILDING SKILLS AND MOTIVATION

Margaret H. Sibley

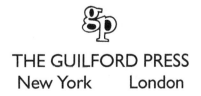

THE GUILFORD PRESS
New York   London

Copyright © 2017 The Guilford Press
A Division of Guilford Publications, Inc.
370 Seventh Avenue, Suite 1200, New York, NY 10001
www.guilford.com

Printed in the United States of America

This book is printed on acid-free paper.

Last digit is print number: 9   8   7   6   5   4   3

The author has checked with sources believed to be reliable in her efforts to provide information that
is complete and generally in accord with the standards of practice that are accepted at the time of
publication. However, in view of the possibility of human error or changes in behavioral, mental health,
or medical sciences, neither the author, nor the editors and publisher, nor any other party who has been
involved in the preparation or publication of this work warrants that the information contained herein
is in every respect accurate or complete, and they are not responsible for any errors or omissions or the
results obtained from the use of such information. Readers are encouraged to confirm the information
contained in this book with other sources.

Library of Congress Cataloging-in-Publication Data
Names: Sibley, Margaret H., author.
Title: Parent–teen therapy for executive function deficits and ADHD :
    building skills and motivation / Margaret H. Sibley.
Description: New York : The Guilford Press, [2017] | Includes bibliographical
    references and index.
Identifiers: LCCN 2016010794 | ISBN 9781462527694 (pbk. : alk. paper)
Subjects: | MESH: Attention Deficit Disorder with Hyperactivity—therapy |
    Adolescent | Executive Function | Parent–Child Relations | Family
    Therapy—methods
Classification: LCC RJ506.H9 | NLM WS 350.8.A8 | DDC 616.85/8900835—dc23
LC record available at *http://lccn.loc.gov/2016010794*

About the Author

Margaret H. Sibley, PhD, is Assistant Professor of Psychiatry and Behavioral Health in the Herbert Wertheim College of Medicine at Florida International University, where she conducts research on the assessment and treatment of adolescents and adults with attention-deficit/hyperactivity disorder. A clinical psychologist and member of the Motivational Interviewing Network of Trainers, Dr. Sibley works closely with community mental health agencies and schools to enhance professional practices for teens and families. She has written numerous journal articles on ADHD and has been the principal investigator on several studies evaluating how to engage families of teens in successful therapy. Dr. Sibley is a recipient of the Young Scientist Award from Children and Adults with Attention-Deficit/Hyperactivity Disorder (CHADD) and of fellowships from the Klingenstein Third Generation Foundation and the American Psychological Foundation, among other honors.

Preface

It's the early evening on a day in mid-August 2009. I am standing on a grass soccer field trying inconspicuously to check the time on my watch. Mrs. Marshall[1] has been trying to catch my ear for a few days to talk about her son Brendan. Out of the corner of my eye, I see her making a beeline toward me. Brendan is in my care at a summer camp for teens with attention-deficit/hyperactivity disorder (ADHD). The focus of this camp is teaching organization and planning skills to teens and intensively turning these skills into habits through daily practice and reinforcement. This was Brendan's third summer at our camp. During the first 2 years, he was often in detention for misbehavior, rarely showed effort during activities, and had a penchant for mischief. This year, he had turned it around and was making unexpected strides at camp.

Mrs. Marshall approached from my right side and began to talk rapidly about her desire to continue Brendan's progress. She anxiously anticipated the day 3 weeks ahead when he would return to school. Mrs. Marshall wanted to know if I would continue to work with Brendan on a weekly basis when camp came to a close. I had grown accustomed to this request. I usually apologized to parents and said that I was unavailable. I knew from personal experience that weekly therapy with families like the Marshalls involved a lot of parent–teen conflict, being told as a therapist that my suggestions were useless, and a variety of other roadblocks to convincing parents and teens to try something new. But this time, I said yes.

The common story told to me by parents in these after-camp encounters was that the community lacked weekly therapy options that were well tailored to their

---

[1]This book contains case presentations that are derived from composites of clients. All client information has been disguised to protect the identities of the individuals.

teens. Some parents complained that therapists were treating teens using approaches that were more appropriate for younger children. Many remarked that relevant skills (e.g., organization, time management, planning) were not taught in talk therapy or that parents were not included in counseling sessions. Most expressed that it was difficult to find parenting resources on navigating the life of a struggling teen.

I agreed to Mrs. Marshall's request because, in quiet moments between basketball games, study halls, water balloon fights, and therapy groups, I began to imagine a once-weekly treatment that might better serve teens like Brendan. I wanted to borrow skill modules from our summer program, train parents to monitor and reinforce skill practice, and help parents advocate for partnership with the school to promote school-based skill practice.

After several unsuccessful attempts to treat families like the Marshalls, I finally had a clear sense of the population-specific engagement issues that prevented uptake of therapy skills. Motivation problems in teens required adult oversight to promote teen skill use, yet many parents seemed unwilling or unable to consistently monitor and reinforce teen behavior. Some parents we worked with harbored beliefs about their teens that interfered with treatment delivery, assuming their teenagers were incapable of independent work, therefore requiring high levels of parental assistance and contradicting their belief that an adolescent was too old for parental supervision. Some parents emphatically stated that contingency management was thoroughly ineffective ("I've taken everything away and it doesn't affect his behavior at all!"). Teens also often presented as disheartened and uninterested in participating in treatment. I did not blame them—spending an hour talking with a therapist and parent about your problems was not exactly fun.

By midsummer, I had a spiral-bound notebook full of ideas for the new treatment program. We needed to integrate our skills-based approach within a framework that would empower parents and teens to explore their goals and values, increase openness to trying new ways of doing things at home, make and sustain changes for their own reasons, and see the possibility of success with their own eyes. Most of all, I desired an approach that instilled and maintained hope in families like the Marshalls.

Everyone always said that for work with difficult-to-engage clients, motivational interviewing (MI) should be used. In 2009, I did not know much about MI. Searching for engagement strategies to integrate into my burgeoning treatment idea, I saw the second edition of *Motivational Interviewing* (Miller & Rollnick, 2002) on the bookshelf of a coworker and asked to borrow it. I absorbed its content over a rainy weekend and felt like I had finally found the missing piece of my treatment. I probably filled a dozen pages in my spiral notebook that weekend. By Monday, it was all coming together.

This new integrated approach to treating teens with ADHD was clunky at first. I have a lot of gratitude for the early families, like the Marshalls, who patiently allowed us to work out our vision for this program. It turns out that folding together active components of several treatments in a way that produces one coherent whole is very challenging. We wanted to incorporate elements of family therapy, behavioral parent training, organization skills training, and MI. Over 6 years of work with hundreds of families, we slowly addressed questions about module content and sequencing. Through a lot of trial and error, our team members helped each other find the heart of MI in our skills-based approach. Some of these team members to whom I feel forever grateful for their collaboration, insight, and contributions are Paulo Graziano, Tuma Kuriyan, Karen Derefinko, and Elizabeth Taquechel. Countless graduate students have also given their time and energy to delivering and scrutinizing this treatment. Each of them contributed something unique and important to the approach described herein.

This treatment is indebted to leaders in our field who conceptualized and developed the four approaches integrated in this book. Early in my training I read Gerald Patterson and Marion Forgatch's book *Parents and Adolescents Living Together* (Forgatch & Patterson, 1989) on a long airplane ride. The ideas in this book helped frame the parent–teen collaborative therapy approach presented in this treatment. I was fortunate to receive graduate training from Steven Evans, a developer of organization skills training for ADHD, and William Pelham, a leader in the field of behavioral parent training. The skills this program provides to parents and teens are largely drawn from these approaches. MI is the glue of this treatment. The work of William Miller, Stephen Rollnick, and their colleagues has inspired me to prioritize warmth, compassion, and client empowerment in a skills-based approach that has been historically didactic. Whenever I spend time with the welcoming and synergistic community of the Motivational Interviewing Network of Trainers (MINT), I leave dozens of pages deeper into an ink-drenched notebook, with so much to think about. In my relatively short time as a member of this group, I have come to understand the therapeutic profession in a completely new light.

After half a decade developing this treatment in a university clinic, I felt called to bring it to the community of mental health professionals in my hometown of Miami, Florida. I wanted their scrutiny. I wanted them to tell me all the ways my approach would not work for their patients. I wanted them to help me make the program more accessible. They taught me how to describe the approach in ways that better relate to clinicians who work in the trenches. They gave me honest feedback on aspects of treatment that felt too academic or mechanistic. They also shared with me valuable strategies that they found worked in their decades of experience with families. I have so much respect and gratitude for these professionals—particularly my colleagues at the Institute for Child and Family Health, Switchboard of Miami, Psych Solutions, Inc., and Miami–Dade County Public Schools.

I always wanted to chronicle our approach in a book that could serve as a reference to therapists who relate to the struggle of finding an appropriate strategy for working with these families. Because thousands of minds are better than just a few, I hope readers will pick up the development of this program where we left off—using what we have figured out so far as a way to organize their thoughts on where to go next. Putting experiences into words that connect with people is challenging. I reached out to a range of individuals who I thought could help me stay on the right track and, in return, received more helpful feedback and serious attention than I ever expected. I am so thankful to the following individuals for reading sections of this book and providing me with honest and thoughtful feedback: Paulo Graziano, Tuma Kuriyan, Candace Morley, Pablo Martin, Elizabeth Taquechel, Fran Wymbs, Amy Altszuler, Annie Morrow, Rob Ogle, Raquel Melendez, Nillie Fallah, Jen Connison, Karen McCormick, Lourdes Rodriguez, and Analay Perez. The biggest thank-you goes to Kitty Moore and the team at The Guilford Press for guiding me through the new experience of creating a book for public consumption. I learned so much from absorbing their expertise about how to connect with an audience.

Finally, a majority of this book was written under the clear blue skies, crisp mountain air, and dolomite limestone cliffs of Ten Sleep, Wyoming. I am thankful to that town for providing the conditions I needed to produce a lot of text in a limited period of time. Thank-you also to Robert Salom for agreeing to go climbing with me every day at 3 o' clock if I had written at least 10 good pages.

Contents

1. Attention, Executive Functioning, and Motivation Problems in Teens   1

What's Really Going On with Marcus?   3

Navigating Adolescence   5

Finding Success in Adolescence   8

How to Help   9

Engaging Parents as Stakeholders   11

Overcoming Negative Parenting Patterns   11

Long-Term Success   13

Treatment Model   15

Empirical Support   16

2. Overview of STAND   18

An Integrated Approach   18

Session Structure   19

Materials   22

Who Can Deliver STAND?   23

Who Is Age Appropriate?   24

Who Can Be the Participating Parent?   25

Selecting and Prioritizing Treatment Goals   26

Addressing Comorbidities   26

How Much Change Is Expected?   28

Booster Sessions to Maintain Change   29

Delivering Treatment in a Group   29

This Book   30

3. **Case Conceptualization**   33

Family-Informed Case Conceptualization   33

Assessment Philosophy: Consideration of Both Strengths and Difficulties   34

Sources of Information   34

Recommended Measures   35

Case Impressions   37

Presenting Case Impressions in Engagement Module 1   38

Finalizing Case Conceptualization   39

Creating Change Cards   39

Using Case Conceptualization to Focus Treatment   45

    Rating Scale 3.1. Adolescent Academic Problems Checklist (AAPC)   47

    Rating Scale 3.2. Parent Academic Management Scale (PAMS)   49

4. **Motivational Interviewing in STAND**   51

The Case for MI in STAND   52

The MI Spirit in STAND   53

Resolving Parent and Teen Ambivalence   55

Core MI Skills   56

MI in STAND Sessions   64

MI Training and Integrity   64

5. **Engagement Modules**   67

Engagement Module 1: Understanding the Family   68

Engagement Module 2: Focusing Treatment Goals   80

Engagement Module 3: Partnership Skills   89

Engagement Module 4: Creating Structure at Home   97

    Worksheet 5.1. What's Important to Me Right Now?   104

    Worksheet 5.2. Strengths and Areas of Difficulty   105

    Worksheet 5.3. Parenting Patterns   106

    Worksheet 5.4. Parenting History   107

    Worksheet 5.5 (Parent). Home Exercise: Into the Future   108

    Worksheet 5.5 (Teen). Home Exercise: Into the Future   109

    Worksheet 5.6. Personal Goals   110

    Worksheet 5.7. STAND Menu   111

    Worksheet 5.8 (Parent). Home Exercise: Letter from the Future   112

    Worksheet 5.8 (Teen). Home Exercise: Letter from the Future   113

    Worksheet 5.9. Staying Calm   114

    Worksheet 5.10. Commmunication Skills   115

    Worksheet 5.11. Planning a Parent–Teen Meeting   116

Worksheet 5.12. Current Structure at Home   117

Worksheet 5.13. Parent–Teen Contract   118

6. **Skill Modules**   119

Structure of the Universal Skill Module   120

Skill Module 1: Writing Down Homework   129

Skill Module 2: Making a Homework Plan   132

Skill Module 3: Organization Checkups   136

Skill Module 4: Time Management Strategies   141

Skill Module 5: Study Skills   146

Skill Module 6: Note Taking   151

Skill Module 7: Problem Solving   155

Worksheet 6.1. Writing Down Homework Practice Plan   160

Worksheet 6.2. Writing Down Homework Contract   161

Worksheet 6.3. Homework Practice Plan   162

Worksheet 6.4. Homework Contract   163

Worksheet 6.5. Staying Organized   164

Worksheet 6.6. Sample Organization Checkup Practice Plan   165

Worksheet 6.7. Organization Checkup Practice Plan   166

Worksheet 6.8. Organization Contract   167

Worksheet 6.9. How to Break Down Tasks to Get Started   168

Worksheet 6.10. Sample Homework List   169

Worksheet 6.11. Time Management Contract   170

Worksheet 6.12. Active Studying   171

Worksheet 6.13. Flash Cards   172

Worksheet 6.14. Fake Word Activity: Flash Cards   173

Worksheet 6.15. Notes from Text   174

Worksheet 6.16. Study Plan   175

Worksheet 6.17. Note-Taking Practice Sheet   176

Worksheet 6.18. Note-Taking Contract   177

Worksheet 6.19. Problem Solving   178

Worksheet 6.20. Home Contract Template   179

7. **Mobilizing Modules**   180

Mobilizing Module 1: Engaging the School   181

Mobilizing Module 2: Habit Formation   187

Mobilizing Module 3: Making an Action Plan   193

Mobilizing Module 4: Keeping Momentum   199

Worksheet 7.1. How Can My School Help?   207

Worksheet 7.2. Menu of Strategies to Engage School Staff   208

Worksheet 7.3. School Conversation   209
Worksheet 7.4. Next Steps   210
Worksheet 7.5. Toolbox   211
Worksheet 7.6. Building a Daily Routine   212
Worksheet 7.7. Action Plan Ideas   213
Worksheet 7.8. Action Plan   214
Worksheet 7.9. Action Plan Log   215
Worksheet 7.10. Next Steps   216

8. Clinical Advice   217

Disengagement   217
Session Management   219
Parental Interference   223
Troubleshooting Home Structure   226
Additional Interfering Factors   229
Termination   231

References   233

Index   235

Purchasers of this book can download and print the rating scales and worksheets
at *www.guilford.com/sibley-forms* for personal use or use with individual clients.

CHAPTER 1

Attention, Executive Functioning, and Motivation Problems in Teens

The phone alarm goes off at 6:00 A.M., then again at 6:15, and at 6:30, without Marcus stirring. It is not until 6:45, when his mother pounds on his bedroom door, that he begins to gain consciousness. His mother yells, "The bus comes in five minutes." She has a critical meeting at work she cannot afford to miss. "You have to catch the bus," she tells him frantically, "I can't be late to work again because I had to drop you off at school."

Marcus stumbles out of bed and stares at the mess around his room. His shoes, textbooks, soccer equipment, and laptop cover the floor. His phone alarm chimes repetitively as he sifts about his belongings, trying to put a stop to the noise. He thought he had just had the phone in his hand a minute ago. Mom pounds the door again and rattles the locked doorknob. Increasingly upset, her tone escalates: "Marcus, I can't do this again. Unlock this door right now."

He bursts out 4 minutes later, with no time for breakfast, brushing his teeth, gathering his textbooks, or having a moment to think about what happened to the end-of-term math assignment he needs that day for class. Marcus catches the bus today, his final Monday of eighth grade, but barely. And his important assignment lies underneath his bed, kicked aside when he was playing video games the night before.

The bell for first period rings. Marcus gazes longingly over his shoulder at the popular group of students in his class, chatting, laughing, likely with their assignments safely stowed in their backpacks. He slowly makes his way to his seat in the middle of the classroom. His teacher instructs the class to turn in the math assignment. Marcus unzips his backpack and digs through the mishmash of papers hunting for his assignment. He's sure he finished it last night. Where was it? He quickly texts his mother: "What did you do with my math assignment?!" Exasperated, he notices his teacher standing next to his desk. The rule of no texting in class means his phone is about to be confiscated.

"I wasn't really texting! I was just trying to figure out why my mom took my math assignment out of my bag." His protest falls on deaf ears. The phone is confiscated, and his fellow classmates snicker something about his mommy from the back of the room. He blushes. The teacher begins to review material for the final exam. Marcus may have heard her voice, but he focuses his attention on the activity outside the classroom window, watching high-schoolers dribble a soccer ball down the field. When the teacher announces the homework assignment, Marcus's mind is far away, counting the number of days until the start of the World Cup.

Back home after school, Marcus calls his mother from their home phone to explain his cell phone confiscation. He demands that she stop at school on her way home from work to pick up the phone and complain to the principal, expressing his conviction that the teacher was picking on him. He believes that the teacher always unfairly assumes he was doing something wrong. When Marcus hangs up the phone, he opens the cupboard, finds an unopened bag of chips, and turns on the television. *Wait, was there math homework?* he wonders. He doesn't remember any. Probably just to study for the test, but he knows it isn't until Thursday, so he has time to study tomorrow. Plus, he wants to catch up on episodes of one of his favorite shows before his mother returns from work and starts nagging him to do homework. She'd better get his phone back tonight, he thinks, fiddling with the casing of the TV remote.

Two hours later, Marcus's mother opens the front door and drops a thick file folder on the kitchen table. She pours a glass of red wine and walks into the living room. She fixes her gaze on Marcus, who is sprawled on the couch with his eyes glued to the television. He turns to her. "Did you get my phone back?" Angrily, she replies, "I went all the way to school to catch someone before it closed. I found your counselor in the office and asked her about your phone. She didn't know anything about it. But she knew all about the 10 detentions you received this month and how you didn't show up to serve any of them. What is going on?"

Marcus ignores her demands for an explanation and focuses only on his phone. "You didn't get my phone!?" His mind returns to and then fixates on his teacher's unfairness. "She had no right to take away my phone. It's stealing. I'm going to complain about her to the school board. This is injustice." As Marcus's mother steers the conversation back to his detentions, he refuses to let up on his complaints about the teacher. "She gave me those detentions for no reason. She is targeting me." The discussion continues in this manner for 10 minutes, with Marcus blaming his teacher and his mother demanding answers about the detentions. Finally, she retreats to her bedroom and closes the door firmly behind her. Marcus turns back to the television and reaches back into his bag of chips, lifting a handful to his mouth as he settles back into his show. At 1:00 in the morning he sleepily drags himself to bed, setting his alarm to go off 5 hours later.

The evening caps what appears to be a very unlucky and stressful day for a teenager—yet for Marcus, this Monday represents a relatively typical day in his life.

What's Really Going On with Marcus?

Most therapists who treat teenagers have met Marcus. He may be a typically developing teen who stumbles with the increasing demands of adolescence. He may have a clinical diagnosis of attention deficit/hyperactivity disorder (ADHD), an autism spectrum disorder (ASD), or another diagnosable neurocognitive deficit. What is clear is that Marcus struggles in a way that significantly affects his daily life. Marcus could benefit from intervention—but which approach would be best for him?

There are several treatment modalities that target the types of problems Marcus experiences. However, each approach tends to target just a single aspect of his impairments. Marcus and his mother easily spiral into stressful arguments when he fails to meet his mother's expectations. Traditional family therapy approaches may create positive communication and strengthen the parent–teen relationship, but they don't treat other issues that underlie the problem, such as his lack of organization, time management, and planning skills that create major problems with completion of homework and his daily routine and thereby contribute to tension with his mother. Organization skills training approaches teach teens strategies to better manage their schoolwork and daily activities; however, to promote independent skill use, the parent typically must provide structure at home that motivates the teen to practice skills daily. Marcus's mother relies on an exhausting combination of reminding, lecturing, and yelling to extract effort from Marcus, which may help him do his work but can damage their relationship, increase parental mental health problems, and stifle Marcus's independence. Behavioral parent training can offer Marcus's mother skills in using contingencies to motivate him to complete daily tasks independently; however, failing to involve Marcus in this process can stifle teen autonomy and undermine his engagement in behavioral interventions. Finally, Marcus holds several maladaptive beliefs that negatively influence his behavior—namely, that completing schoolwork is boring and that his teacher is out to get him. Cognitive-behavioral therapy may help Marcus challenge these thoughts to decrease procrastination and improve his emotional reaction to stressful situations, but again it won't address the entire picture.

In sum, each of these treatments may enhance functioning in one domain; yet the difficulties Marcus experiences are not discrete. Problems with homework and school behavior lead him to argue with his mother. Maladaptive cognitions trigger problems with his teacher and arguments with his mother. Poor planning affects his school grades. His mother's lack of structure at home exacerbates Marcus's disorganization and motivation problems. Her tendency to argue back to Marcus further seeds tension in their relationship. When Marcus's mother gives in to his demands, he learns that becoming angry will lead his mother to retreat. With decreased supervision, Marcus's organization and motivation further deteriorate. With teens like Marcus, a one-dimensional approach to treatment can be grossly insufficient.

Some refer to Marcus with terms such as *lazy, inconsiderate, irresponsible, scatterbrained,* or *stupid.* His neuropsychological profile tells a different story. Work by researchers show us that teens like Marcus, who struggle to organize, plan, and self-regulate, often experience developmental deficits in one or more distinct but intertwined neurocognitive processes: attention, executive functioning (EF), and motivation (Barkley, 2014; Castellanos, Sonuga-Barke, Milham, & Tannock, 2006; Sonuga-Barke, 2002). These functions combine to produce goal-directed behavior and involve several regions of the brain, including the prefrontal cortex, striatum, anterior cingulate cortex, and thalamus.

In any given environment, attentional processes determine the brain's selection of particular information for processing. In selection, the brain acknowledges certain pieces of information but passes over others. When Marcus attends to the soccer players outside of his classroom window, his brain ignores the classroom lecture. This selective attention obviously leads to problems for teens such as Marcus when they fail to retain information presented in class or listen to adults who are speaking with them.

EF represents cognitive processes that control effort and behavior. EF is associated with the ability to organize and carry out goal-directed behavior, which includes organizing, planning, holding information in mind, and inhibiting actions that fail to support one's goal. EF also includes functions that provide top-down regulation of the attentional processes just described. Marcus shows impaired EF in a number of areas, including his difficulties keeping track of schoolwork, his tendency to lose materials, his difficulty remembering details, his inability to inhibit emotional verbalizations to adults, and his trouble in carrying out multistep tasks. Magnetic resonance imaging (MRI) scans of Marcus's brain might show less development than those of his classmates in certain areas—most likely in his prefrontal cortex (Shaw et al., 2006), which is the operation center for these functions.

Marcus also shows dysfunction in motivation processes. He experiences delay aversion, which is an atypical level of mental discomfort experienced during unstimulating activities. To escape this discomfort, he gravitates toward immediately gratifying activities, be they emotionally or visually stimulating (e.g., watching soccer out the window, television viewing, video games). His brain cues automatically to distractions that relieve the discomfort of sustaining the mental effort required to focus on uninteresting or difficult tasks. Unfortunately, this inclination to attend only to immediately stimulating activities often prevents him from completing multicomponent tasks and projects that feel hard or boring in the short term. As a result, Marcus chooses to watch television or play video games instead of completing academic tasks that he dreads but that yield important long-term payoffs (e.g., studying for a test, taking the time to clean up his bedroom). During the teen years, many of Marcus's peers will learn to work steadily on multistep assignments, recognizing the long-term gratification of a high grade, college acceptance, or fostering trusting relationships with adults. Instead of being viewed as someone who will "get the job done," Marcus may come to be viewed as inconsistent and unreliable. For Marcus, overcoming motivation problems will be a slow and challenging process.

If brain functioning is disrupted in any of the processes described above, the teen is likely to experience difficulties in self-regulation and enacting goal-directed behavior. For example, a student may receive a poor grade on a homework assignment because he or she cannot force him- or herself to get started or to keep working (motivation problems), has trouble attending to information or instructions needed to complete the assignment correctly (attention problems), or loses the assignment before turning it in (EF problems). Many teens who have problems with one of these functions also have problems with the others. Without recognition and treatment, these deficits may leave a lasting mark that limits their future opportunities.

Navigating Adolescence

The adolescent period is meant to be fun, socially enjoyable, and personally formative (Steinberg, 2010). Adolescence is a time for personal exploration, skill development, building autonomy, and formulating one's own goals. For the first time, teens are given opportunities to organize their daily schedules, tailor their education, and engage in unsupervised peer activities. Teens start to develop their own taste in music and media and passions for sports teams and social causes. And for the first time, they begin to develop more adult-like social relationships. Decisions made and interests forged during the teen years pave the course of adulthood.

All teens possess unique strengths that can be cultivated during the period of adolescence to prepare them for adulthood and for an emotionally healthy and satisfying life. Although we've focused on Marcus's deficits, he also has strengths. He has been a gifted soccer player since elementary school. His interest in video games has allowed him to connect with a range of peers through live multiplayer gaming. As clinicians, we want to recognize his strengths and work with him with the hope that he will reach the milestones of adolescence and create a personally gratifying adult existence. We want Marcus to explore identity within the safety of his teen environment, to independently develop adaptive skills to allow him to leave home in an age-appropriate time frame, and to identify personal goals that guide him toward a positive future. Additionally, we want to make sure that Marcus's deficits do not lead to serious events that may derail his course toward happy and healthy adult living.

Unfortunately, positive adolescent development often eludes individuals like Marcus who display neurocognitive deficits in attention, EF, or motivation. Instead, adolescence may become a challenging period with lasting negative consequences. Social and academic demands increase exponentially in the teen years, and adolescents like Marcus may be unprepared to meet these challenges. We expect teens to independently manage their academic lives, responsibly moderate their use of social media, engage in a range of extracurricular activities, and increasingly contribute to their households and communities. With deficits that interfere with the ability to plan, organize, and self-regulate, teens like Marcus may find the transition to adolescence to be overwhelming.

The secondary school environment is much more complex than elementary school. Teens must independently transition between classes with separate teachers, keep track of assigned work and deadlines, and complete multistep tasks and projects with minimal adult support. Even typically developing teens will at first struggle with academics when adapting to new secondary school environments (Eccles, 2004). However, gradually the foundational skills built in elementary school will successfully carry new middle school students through this rocky transition. Unfortunately, teens with neurocognitive deficits not only naturally struggle with independent self-management but also may have lost years of childhood skill development in less demanding elementary school environments (e.g., lower class placements, failure to participate in after-school activities). With missed opportunities to engage and develop their already lagging EF skills (i.e., organization, time management, planning), these teens may be substantially unprepared for the adolescent transition. Just when teenagers need all of their EF faculties working together, those with neurocognitive challenges have little ability to deal with the increasing complexity of their academic and social lives.

Struggles to independently manage the new demands of adolescence may leave some teens vulnerable to even more serious problems. We know from the work of B. J. Casey and colleagues (Casey, Jones, & Hare, 2008) that the typical adolescent brain experiences uneven development in the systems involved with behavioral decision making. Regions that create pleasure during enjoyable activities (largely through release of the neurotransmitter dopamine) develop earlier than the EF regions that help us to say "no" to behaviors that may at first be pleasurable but that ultimately lead to negative consequences (such as eating too many potato chips or playing video games instead of doing homework). For adolescents, this exaggerated and uninhibited dopamine release excites the teen in the presence of socially or emotionally salient stimuli (e.g., peer attention, social media, romantic encounters, fast driving, substance use). Unfortunately, immature EF regions are unprepared to sufficiently rein in these powerful reward responses. As a result, most teens, whether or not they have EF deficits, are prone to engage in exciting, fun activities that unfortunately can sometimes lead to negative results.

The typical afflictions of adolescence hit hardest when a teen experiences attention problems, EF deficits, motivation problems, or, worse, all three. Adolescent impulses can be difficult for a typical youth to manage, but teens with motivation problems will find these urges even more irresistible. These youth have two biological reasons to engage in risky or irresponsible behavior: (1) an adolescent drive toward emotionally rewarding experience and (2) deficits in motivation that drive them away from monotonous tasks and strengthen a desire to engage in immediately gratifying activities. When EF abilities are underdeveloped compared with those of peers, a teen has the worst of both worlds. With weakened abilities to inhibit impulses, teens with EF deficits can become hamstrung by developmental surges in dopamine. With trouble finding success at home and school and a thirst for immediate gratification, these teens are at highest risk for school disengagement, problems with parents, and participation in problematic activities.

Developmental risk models (Sher, Grekin, & Williams, 2005; Zucker, 2006) warn that major negative life events disrupt adolescent milestones or present serious setbacks in adulthood. These include failure to complete high school or an equivalent vocational certificate, incarceration, addiction, driver's license revocation, severe mental illness, teen pregnancy, major injury, and dependence on government assistance programs. Pathways to many of these negative events begin with school failure and alienation from family members in early adolescence (see Figure 1.1). Many adolescents who fail to find personally rewarding experiences in positive environments— such as extracurricular activities, recreational interests, academics, or prosocial relationships—often seek stimulation from deviant peers, substances, rule breaking, and other risky activities. Not only can these alternatives present imminent negative consequences for the teen, but the absence of positive teen experiences also prevents development of adaptive interests, skills, and identity.

All of Marcus's deficits in attention, EF, and motivation create difficulty with his ability to self-regulate. This problem puts him at risk for school failure (through

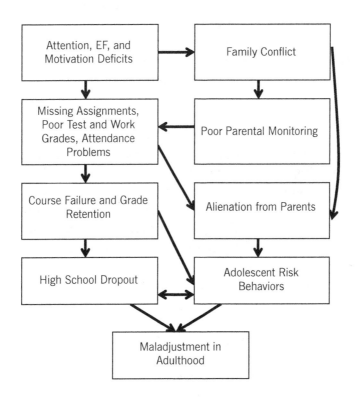

FIGURE 1.1. Pathways to adult maladjustment.

disorganization, disengagement, and poor work completion) and family conflict (through inconsistent completion of responsibilities, behavior problems, and poor verbal self-control that lead to conflicts with parents). For teens with these neuropsychological deficits, the unfolding consequences of academic failure and family stress are further compounded by poor behavioral inhibition. As they struggle to suppress particularly strong urges, these teens are prone to try substances, engage in unprotected sex, disregard rules, and engage in risky driving at higher rates than their peers. The capstone of these pathways is often a teen who drops out of high school. This leads to further problems, as teens who fail to earn degrees by young adulthood will struggle to sustain employment and achieve financial independence. In addition, they may experience severe mental illnesses or may turn to a life of persistent substance abuse and criminal behavior. Thus, due to cascading risks, teens with attention, EF, and motivation deficits are particularly prone to a disrupted adolescence with potentially debilitating consequences by young adulthood (for empirical support for these processes, see Barkley, Murphy, & Fischer, 2008).

Finding Success in Adolescence

To get teens with attention, EF, or motivation problems back on track developmentally requires scaffolding. To achieve critical milestones—identity building, goal formation, skill development, and self-sufficiency— intermediate steps must be set in place. Attempts to permanently remediate teens' underlying neurobiology through cognitive training programs or medication have been largely unsuccessful. So far, the outcomes of brain training programs for this age group reveal that teens master computer practice tasks but that these improvements do not translate into real-world gains (Gray et al., 2012; Steiner, Sheldrick, Gotthelf, & Perrin, 2011). Central nervous system stimulant medications that alter neurochemistry (e.g., Ritalin, Adderall, Concerta, Vyvanse) improve neurocognitive functioning only when the pill is active in the teen's system—improvements reverse once medication wears off (Greenhill et al., 2002). Chronic use of stimulant medications also causes limitations. Over time, physiological tolerance to these drugs' therapeutic effects may suppress their effectiveness (Swanson et al., 1999). In fact, most teens who are prescribed stimulant medications in childhood ask to stop taking the pills in adolescence due to uncomfortable side effects or to the social and self-concept implications of relying on daily medication (for more information on the long-term effects of stimulant medications, see the adolescent results of the Multimodal Treatment Study of Children with ADHD [MTA study]; Molina et al., 2009). Without a way to permanently alter neuropsychological capacities, teens with attention, EF, or motivation deficits must develop *compensatory* skills. For these teens, this becomes a central goal of adolescence: development of long-term strategies for overcoming neurocognitive deficits.

A second goal for teens with attention, motivation, or EF problems is to discover environments that maximize their strengths while minimizing the influence of deficits. Thus a strength-based approach is particularly critical for teens who repeatedly experience failures. These efforts include choosing an educational path that engages the teen (minimizing motivation problems) and turns proclivities into unique skills that will serve the teen in the future. The experience of success in one domain can bring success in others; if Marcus excels on his school soccer team, he will be more appreciated by his peers. He also may push through motivation difficulties during homework to maintain an adequate grade point average (GPA) for team membership. Conversely, environments that are poorly suited to a teen with attention, EF, and motivation problems may increase the daily routine's averseness. This may include academic environments that demand high levels of self-sufficiency (exacerbating the effects of attention and EF deficits), schools with prevalent bullying, classrooms with teachers who are impatient with student symptoms, or highly rigorous academic programs.

Finally, a critical goal for these teens is avoidance of negative life events that disrupt the path to healthy and independent living. As such, deliberate efforts must occur to measuredly increase independence in such a way that requires teens with attention, EF, and motivation deficits to prove readiness for new freedoms. Educational completion is emphasized here. A number of teens with these difficulties fail to finish high school (Barkley et al., 2008), making this outcome one of the most imminent and concerning for these youth. Failure typically begins with incomplete work and poor test grades. Without proper supports, school problems may escalate to course failure, grade retention, and complete disengagement from school (see Figure 1.2).

How to Help

What tools exist for professionals seeking to help teens with attention, EF, and motivation deficits? How does one facilitate identification and development of

---

Key Goals of Adolescence

- Identity formation
- Skill development
- Goal setting
- Self-sufficiency
- Limit testing and experiential learning

Additional Goals for Teens with Deficits

- Developing compensatory strategies
- Identifying environments that maximize strengths and minimize deficits
- Avoiding major negative life events

FIGURE 1.2. Developmental goals of adolescence.

compensatory skills, create opportunities for teens to explore values and interests, and enact measures to prevent major negative life events? Many therapists, counselors, and educators find that professional tools that support these goals are limited. Our field's recognition of the intertwined effects of teen attention, EF, and motivation deficits is fairly recent. Although several one-dimensional approaches to treatment are available to clinicians, integrated approaches for treating these teens are scarce. Several components of treatment must be incorporated to appropriately address the multiple areas of difficulty experienced by these youth.

First, teens need introduction to compensatory skills that help them overcome the effects of their neurocognitive deficits. These efforts involve age-appropriate organization, time management, and planning strategies. Instruction in these strategies has most frequently been delivered by school professionals, in after-school programs, or through multiweek summer programs. When teens practice these techniques, their ability to self-manage improves at home and school (Evans, Schultz, DeMars, & Davis, 2011; Langberg, Epstein, Becker, Girio-Herrera, & Vaughn, 2012).

Compensatory skills in organization, time management, and planning require continuous practice to produce mastery and, finally, habitual independent skill use by the adolescent. The biggest impediment to practice and habit development is the adolescent's motivation problems. Enacting compensatory skills takes effort and adds extra steps to the teen's daily routine. Adolescents with motivation problems are likely to find this extra work aversive. To jump-start skill practice and create lasting habits, treatment of EF deficits must be supplemented with treatment of motivation problems. Methods for addressing teen motivation problems are less developed than is treatment for EF skill deficits. In school-age children, parents and teachers are trained to override motivation deficits by administering salient rewards and consequences to children for meeting (or failing to meet) behavioral targets. The child's excitement at the thought of receiving these adult-administered rewards reduces the discomfort of boring or difficult tasks. In adolescence, contingency management takes a new form. Parents and teens are encouraged to collaborate in devising a daily structure that requires the teen to complete responsibilities before accessing enjoyable activities (Forgatch & Patterson, 1989). This structure is best reinforced by an adult in the teen's life who (1) is in daily contact with the teen, (2) can oversee the teen's access to enjoyable activities, and (3) is willing to allow the teen to contribute to planning and contracting as an equal.

When EF skill instruction and age-appropriate contingency management are delivered in concert, teens develop helpful new habits and begin to connect the dots between practicing organization, time management, and planning skills and achieving success. After a few weeks of consistent skill practice, a teen may begin to see an improvement in school grades. If the pride or newly realized benefits of this success outweigh the mental discomfort of practicing the skill, the teen may continue this habit in the absence of an explicit contingency structure at home. Of course, this epiphany likely is not enough to permanently change teen behavior, but it can be a productive first step for the teen.

Engaging Parents as Stakeholders

There are typically two classes of adult stakeholders engaged in the daily life of teens: parents and secondary school staff. For several reasons, parents may be ideal participants in treatment. First, many parents have more available time and resources than secondary school staff, and they obviously have more emotional investment in the teen. Second, parents are sustainable agents of change; school staff members are only available the year the teen is under their supervision. Third, in middle and high school, a large portion of academic work is completed at home, outside of the purview of school staff. Finally, parents who make lasting changes to their own maladaptive parenting behaviors will create much greater change in their adolescent than could occur by any outside resource or school intervention. If Marcus's mother can work with a therapist to find more appropriate ways to encourage independence and respond to his emotional outbursts, it will pay dividends for Marcus in the long term. The first component of this therapeutic support is often building parental engagement and parents' willingness to modify their own behavior in support of teens' success. Though many parents seek treatment in hopes that a therapist can teach or convince the teen to shape up, the deepest therapeutic work often occurs within the parent. Because maladaptive parental behaviors can take several different forms, sustainable treatment of the parent–teen dyad must accommodate individual differences in the parent's presentation.

Overcoming Negative Parenting Patterns

It is well known that consistent monitoring of teen behavior, positive parent–teen relationships, and allowing some teen autonomy are key elements of successful authoritative parenting—the parenting style that fosters best outcomes among adolescents (Steinberg, Lamborn, Dornbusch, & Darling, 1992). It is also known that these parenting practices tend to be disrupted in parents of teens with attention, EF, and motivation deficits (Edwards, Barkley, Laneri, Fletcher, & Metevia, 2001). Coercive parent–youth interactions unfold over time, such that child self-regulation problems lead to parental frustration, which can further exacerbate a child's behavior problems. As a youth's behavior escalates, parents who eventually give up on enforcing consequences teach their children that the more you protest, the more likely an adult will be to give in. By the arrival of adolescence, these patterns may be deeply ingrained, creating high levels of conflict, parental disengagement, overcontrol, or criticism.

As illustrated in recent work from our group (Sibley et al., 2016), negative parent–child cycles can also apply to academics. In a sample of nearly 300 teens with attention, EF, and motivation problems, parents were asked to complete questionnaires about their typical involvement in adolescent academics—with specific attention to how parents managed attention, EF, and motivation problems in their teens. Statistical analysis of parental response patterns indicated the presence of three broad parent management patterns—two of which exposed habits that actually may worsen teen impairments.

First, there were some parents who seemed to be doing things right. Approximately 20% of parents and teens appeared to be engaging in a collaborative approach to managing teen deficits. These parents cooperatively set a home structure with teens, set limits on their freedom, and required accountability for completing schoolwork. Importantly, parents displaying this pattern appeared to have the highest levels of personal well-being. They experienced less emotional distress and fewer physical ailments, presumably due to the stable and calm home environment that stems from a collaborative approach.

A parental control group, formed by about 40% of the sample, represented a first maladaptive pattern. Many of these parents were highly involved in all aspects of teen organization, time management, and planning (though some limited their overinvolvement to homework help). These activities included frequent assisting with and checking of teens' academic work, high levels of contact with teachers, checking the teens' online grade book daily, and reorganizing school materials without their teens' involvement. When parents believe the adolescent is incapable of completing work independently, the parental control strategy offers an effective short-term solution to failing grades (i.e., parents manage academics for the adolescent and grades improve); however, long-term consequences of this approach undermine adolescent independence. Adolescents may learn that dawdling during academic work will encourage parents to offer a high level of assistance—ultimately reducing the amount of time and effort the teen needs to spend on homework. Teens also fail to develop and practice critical compensatory skills when parents manage academics for them. During treatment, we affectionately call these parents the teens' "personal assistants." This pattern can be debilitating to the teen and also highly taxing to the parent. Parents were most likely to enact this strategy when the teen was younger or showed high levels of EF dysfunction. These parents also reported the highest levels of anxiety and health problems in themselves.

A final parental pattern, termed uninvolved, comprised another 40% of parents in the sample; they represented broad disengagement from their teens' academic work. The older the adolescent, and the stronger the adolescent's motivation problems, the more likely the parent was to display the uninvolved pattern. Many parents who displayed the uninvolved pattern reported previously engaging in the parental control pattern. Perhaps years of adolescent EF and motivation problems that were unaltered by parental micromanagement created hopelessness in some parents. If prior attempts to encourage the teen were unsuccessful, these parents may see no value in continued efforts. Parents displaying the uninvolved pattern also reported higher levels of depression.

These study results suggest that a majority of parents of teens with attention, EF, or motivation problems adopt dysfunctional parenting patterns in natural response to adolescent deficits. Unlike the parents of younger children, parents of adolescents have over a decade of experience interacting with their children and forming stable beliefs about the adolescents' abilities. These beliefs are powerful determinants of the parents' behavior and guide their parenting choices. Often, what professionals see as a parenting *problem* has been the parents' only *solution* for years.

Conflicts are particularly prone to arise when control-oriented parents attempt to withdraw support or uninvolved parents begin to increase oversight. In these cases, teens had not been held accountable for any independent work, and when new limits were suddenly placed on them, conflict ensued. In addition, these teens had not been taught the skills or learned the motivation required to transition to independent academics. As a result, families who desire to change rules and expectations at home may require therapist guidance and support to do so successfully.

Long-Term Success

We've seen that treating attention, EF, and motivation problems in teens requires compensatory skill instruction and practice, implementing a contingent daily structure that is supervised by a supportive adult, and remediation of maladaptive parenting problems. Earlier we noted that motivation problems may return when reinforcements for skill practice are removed. So, how does one help teens develop skills to overcome motivation deficits in the long run?

Let us reconsider the nature of teen motivation problems. Teens with motivation deficits, such as delay aversion, experience an unusual level of discomfort with monotony or effortful tasks when there is no immediately foreseeable benefit. This discomfort drives them away from activities that require time or effort with little short-term reward, even when there is high long-term payoff. Motivation problems occur as a function of two factors: time and perceived reward value. Long delays for payoffs reduce the likelihood that the teen will complete the activity or change the behavior. Marcus will be much more likely to study for tomorrow's test than one that is scheduled for next week.

If the teen perceives little benefit to the behavior (low perceived reward value), he or she also is less likely to complete it, even if the payoff is immediate. Marcus may choose not to study for an impending test if he has no interest in improving his GPA or believes that studying will not help his test performance. In teens with motivation problems, dopamine transmission is altered such that an immediate and highly valued benefit to a behavior is often required to overcome the dread of sustained effort. So Marcus may not study for a test unless he decides that studying will accomplish a meaningful goal with immediate payoff.

Thus part of treatment might be a search for natural circumstances that have high reward values to the teen and reduced wait time for payoff. What does this look like? The teen should be encouraged to discover environments that maximize the

<u>presence and frequency of valued natural and adaptive reinforcers</u>. In Marcus's case, this means finding a high school with a strong soccer program, a team that values him, and academic electives that engage his interests.

In addition to maximizing the presence of natural environmental rewards, therapeutic work can strengthen teen response to these built-in contingencies by increasing their perceived value. Marcus may enjoy soccer, but helping him comprehend the benefits of this activity (e.g., building social relationships, physical activity, developing leadership skills, recognition from adults and peers, college acceptance) may strengthen the perceived value of soccer. Marcus may embrace the benefits of soccer but not believe he has the academic ability to qualify for athletic participation. Thus work may also build a teen's self-efficacy, forging beliefs that adaptive behaviors are worthwhile because they are *likely* to lead to desired rewards. Earlier, it was mentioned that one way this can be done is by enacting a contingent structure in the short term that spurs skill use and allows adolescents to witness themselves being successful. During therapy sessions, appropriately processing this initial success can clarify the relationship between hard work, skill use, and successful performance. Exploring the benefits of successful performance (e.g., athletic eligibility, pleasing a parent, higher school grades, increased self-worth) can further strengthen the perceived value of natural rewards associated with teen efforts.

Meanwhile, long-term success for the parent also means therapeutic attention to parent motivational and cognitive factors that maintain maladaptive parenting practices. As part of this process, parents embark on a parallel journey of finding reasons to make and sustain long-term parenting changes (e.g., requiring teens to complete work independently, monitoring and reinforcing teen work completion) by (1) increasing the perceived value of this change (e.g., fostering a positive future for the teen, allowing the parents more time for themselves in the evening, reducing parent–teen conflict, creating academic independence) and (2) building parent self-efficacy—forging beliefs that teen's behavior *can be influenced* with the proper parenting strategies in place.

There is a well-established literature on using therapy to alter aspects of motivation in adults and adolescents. Once such approach is motivational interviewing (MI), a therapeutic paradigm that has undergone decades of refinement (see Miller & Rollnick, 2013). MI supports the treatment goal of strengthening the value of natural rewards for adolescent adaptive behavior (EF skill use, academic effort) and parent changes (reducing control strategies or increasing oversight of academics). MI also supports the treatment goal of building self-efficacy in teens (helping adolescents see that adaptive behavior will lead to receipt of valued natural rewards) and parents (helping parents see that when they change their parenting style, changes in the adolescent's home behavior will follow). MI can accomplish these goals by guiding the client to discuss changes in a way that increases discussion of the positive aspects of change and reduces attention to arguments in favor of the status quo. Chapter 4 provides a full discussion of the use of MI in parent–teen treatment for attention, EF, and motivation problems.

Treatment Model

The preceding discussion highlights the multifaceted challenges facing teens with attention, EF, and/or motivation problems. As such, maximally effective treatment for these teens often requires multifaceted therapy. Attention and EF deficits can be *# 1* targeted by teaching teens compensatory skills. Motivation deficits can be treated in *# 2* the short term through an adult-overseen contingency structure that incites initial teen success—and in the long term by incorporating therapeutic techniques designed to build motivation. Over time, therapy may enhance the perceived value of natural rewards for adaptive behaviors and build adolescent self-efficacy as practiced skills slowly lead to success. Finally, maladaptive parenting processes are addressed in the short term by training parents to appropriately practice reinforcing home structure. In the long term, maintenance of appropriate parenting practices can be encouraged by increasing the perceived value of these parenting changes (see Figure 1.3).

The treatment described herein represents an integrated and developmentally informed approach for teens with attention, EF, and motivation problems. To address the multiple mechanisms of dysfunction in this population (many of whom receive a clinical diagnosis of ADHD, a learning disorder, or an ASD), this approach combines training in compensatory skills, parent–teen collaborative contingency management, and MI. This integrated treatment (which we refer to as Supporting Teens' Autonomy Daily, or STAND for short) is an autonomy support approach that engages parents and teens in age-appropriate and collaborative care. Other treatments for this population may not be integrated—including training only in EF skills, parent behavior management, family communication skills, or cognitive restructuring. STAND seeks to be an accessible approach that helps parents and teens understand how the brain influences behavior (*why* teens have trouble paying attention or controlling impulses) and what steps they must take to find success. STAND's integrated approach frames treatment for any adolescent with significant impairments in attention, EF, or motivation domains—regardless of clinical diagnosis.

general tx structure:

1. Develop compensatory skills.
2. Identify environments that maximize presence and frequency of salient natural rewards.
3. Create an age-appropriate contingency structure by contracting with the parents to overcome short-term motivation problems.
4. Support parents in practicing consistent implementation of adaptive parenting skills.
5. Use MI to increase perceived value of natural rewards in the teen's environment and enhance teen self-efficacy for achieving success (long-term improvement in motivation).
6. Use MI to increase the parents' perceived value of making parenting changes and to enhance parents' self-efficacy for influencing teen behavior (long-term maintenance of parenting practices).

FIGURE 1.3. Treatment goals for adolescents with attention, EF, and motivation problems.

Empirical Support

We began the process of evaluating STAND's efficacy by piloting the treatment with 36 families. To test how STAND compared with typical community resources, half of our sample was randomly assigned to receive STAND while the other half pursued usual care in the community. Parents, teens, and teachers of teens in both groups filled out questionnaires about the teens' functioning before treatment, midway through treatment, and after treatment. We also collected observational measures of the participants' organization skills and school grades.

This first pilot study (Sibley et al., 2013) indicated that therapists found the new approach to be user-friendly, that all families completed treatment, and that nearly 90% of families took the step of scheduling a meeting with the adolescents' schools to discuss integrating home and school treatment approaches. Both parents and teens rated treatment as highly credible—they believed it addressed the problems that initially led them to present for help. Furthermore, both parents and teens reported that they enjoyed working with the therapists. We found these results encouraging given initially high levels of discord in the early didactic version of our program—these data suggested that MI might be helping engagement.

With respect to parental consistency, by the end of treatment, a majority of parents reported daily contingency management to reinforce adolescent skill use. Adolescents reported that the most helpful part of treatment was time spent discussing goals and interests, as well as creating a new structure at home that put responsibilities before enjoyable activities. Parents reported that the most helpful aspects of treatment were skill modules delivered to the adolescent. All families were highly satisfied with treatment.

Our preliminary work with this small group of families suggested that, compared with the community treatment group, adolescents who received STAND used EF strategies with greater frequency, more consistently recorded daily homework assignments, earned higher grades in school, and experienced sizable reductions in inattention and hyperactivity/impulsivity symptoms. In addition, parents reported the reduction in oppositional behavior and conflict at home.

To further test STAND with a larger sample of teens, we conducted a study in which 128 adolescents were randomly assigned to receive the program or a community control condition (Sibley, Graziano, et al., in press). Prior to treatment, after treatment, and 6 months later, parents, adolescents, and teachers provided similar ratings to those in the pilot study. Once again, adolescents who attended treatment made significant improvements in skill use, ADHD symptom severity, and organization skills relative to the community group. These effects were maintained 6 months after treatment ceased (see Figure 1.4).

Taking a closer look at parent changes during treatment, this study revealed that parents who participated in STAND were more likely than those in the community group to set a structure at home that required responsibilities to be completed before enjoyable activities. Most important, compared with parents in the

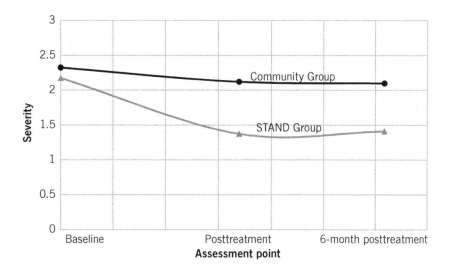

FIGURE I.4. Group differences in organization, time management, and planning problems.

community group, parents who participated in STAND reported lower levels of parenting stress after completing the program. This effect also was maintained 6 months after treatment. Interestingly, to arrive at these positive outcomes, parents made different types of changes—some increased their oversight of the teen's schoolwork and daily responsibilities, whereas others decreased their micromanagement, allowing the teen to take on more independent work. Each family appeared to create its own unique pathway to improve life at home and school.

We are currently conducting additional research to better understand how a treatment such as STAND might best serve families. One study compares STAND delivered in its typical individual parent–teen format with STAND delivered to families in a group setting. Our hope is to understand whether mechanisms of integrated treatment can be engaged in this lower-resource approach. We also recently began piloting STAND delivered via videoconference to families who live too far from our clinic to receive treatment in person. Results thus far are encouraging. Finally, we began an initiative to train community therapists to deliver STAND in community mental health agencies. Our goal is to understand how STAND may be adapted to best serve adolescents receiving treatment in a variety of treatment provision settings.

CHAPTER 2

Overview of STAND

An Integrated Approach

Because the multifaceted deficits of teens with attention, EF, and motivation problems may benefit most from a multicomponent approach to treatment (see Chapter 1), STAND represents an integrated and modular approach. Some therapists find comfort in a circumscribed and step-by-step guide to delivering a treatment program. Other therapists value the leeway to analyze a case and devise a unique treatment plan given the present needs and priorities of a family; these individuals may wish to extract only the components of STAND that seem most relevant to their case, leaving other suggestions behind. To provide a fitting resource to each of these individuals, this book outlines treatment modularly. These modules are packaged neatly for the therapist who appreciates a step-by-step approach. For the therapist who takes an eclectic or constructivist approach to treatment planning, they may be unpacked and spread through treatment as a therapist deems appropriate.

Teens with attention and EF difficulties present with a range of deficits—some struggle with planning, others with time management, and yet others with holding details in mind while completing multistep tasks. Many struggle to inhibit behavioral impulses. Most teens with attention and EF problems present with a number of these difficulties, but there is substantial variability in difficulties across adolescents. As a result, it is not necessary for each family to complete all treatment modules.

Many parents expect that introducing a skill to a teen is all that is necessary to create a new habit, and they may quickly anger and blame the teen when instruction does not lead to adoption. To dismantle this expectation, when skills are introduced in STAND, they are flanked with discussion of changes at home that maximize the likelihood of long-term skill use. This includes how to integrate skills into the teen's daily routine, how the parent can monitor skill use, and how to create structure at home that requires responsibilities to be complete before the teen can engage in enjoyable activities. Sewing seeds for long-term skill maintenance (both for adolescent skill use and positive parenting strategies) can also occur during these discussions. MI (discussed more in Chapter 4) is blended into conversations to help parents and teens carefully process the impact of new behaviors on their daily lives and to promote new beliefs about their abilities. *engagement + mobilizing modules*

Skills-based modules are bookended with engagement and mobilizing modules. Engagement modules prime parent and teen motivation to engage in treatment. Mobilizing modules review lessons learned during treatment and empower parents and teens to make lasting changes in light of treatment experiences. Engagement modules preemptively address teen motivation problems and negative parental beliefs about the teen. These early sessions also encourage parents and teens to reflect on their priorities and goals for the future. Mobilizing modules encourage parents and teens to consider insights they gained during STAND and create a collaborative plan for converting new skills into a daily routine. These sessions utilize MI to strengthen parent and teen commitment to continuing new skills after treatment ceases. An overview of STAND modules appears in Table 2.1 on the next page. These sessions are outlined in detail in Chapters 5–7. *engagement → mobilization*

Session Structure

STAND sessions are optimized when attended by both the teen and his or her primary caretaker (see below). Holding sessions with both family members present emphasizes the collaborative nature of treatment, prevents the misperception that the therapist is differentially aligned with either the parent or teen, and allows the parent and teen to be aware of each other's role in treatment exercises. Sometimes the therapist may decide that an aspect of treatment is better addressed with only the parent or only the teen present—this may be particularly true when discussing parenting problems or personal information that the teen or parent may be uncomfortable disclosing in front of each other.

Sessions are designed to be 1 hour long—fitting within the structure of typical outpatient settings. Of course, a variety of factors, including therapist experience level, the details of a case, and a family's characteristics, can influence the therapist's ability to fully cover all suggested session material. As such, therapists are encouraged to tailor the length of the session to the family and setting.

STAND is intended as a modular treatment with significant individualization within and between sessions. Individualization is enhanced when significant input is garnered from the family. As a result, engagement module 2 is structured to collaboratively design a treatment plan with the family; families review a treatment menu that lists seven skill modules and are encouraged to select from the list with therapist input. In our experience, incorporating too many skill modules successively can overwhelm or overburden the teen and parent. We recommend starting with three and introducing others only when mastery of initial skills is well under way. *3 modules to start!*

TABLE 2.1. Overview of STAND Therapy Modules

Engagement modules

E1: Understanding the Family	Discuss parent and adolescent values and strengths and typical parenting methods. Develop discrepancy between values and current behavior. Strengthen commitment to improved functioning. Discuss goals for future. *review of assessments*
E2: Focusing Treatment Goals	Identify and prioritize parent and adolescent areas for change. Select potential treatment modules using treatment menu. Identify treatment goals. Write letter from future self.
E3: Partnership Skills	Discuss staying calm in stressful situations. Introduce reflective listening skills and "I" statements. Make a plan for holding a parent–teen meeting at home to practice skills.
E4: Creating Structure at Home	Discuss structure that balances responsibilities and enjoyable activities at home. Discuss how structure that puts responsibilities first can build motivation and independence. Introduce skill of using a parent–teen contract to make a plan at home.

Skill modules

S1: Writing Down Homework	Discuss current attempts to remember homework. Strengthen commitment to remember homework. Make a plan for recording homework (with parent monitoring and contract).
S2: Making a Homework Plan	Discuss current homework habits and goals for homework completion. Strengthen commitment to improve homework completion. Create plan for homework time with parent monitoring component. Implement parent–teen homework contract.
S3: Organization Checks	Discuss current organization habits and goals. Strengthen commitment to improve organization. Establish organization system (for book bag, bedroom, etc.) and document on checklist. Establish parent–teen contract for monitoring organization.
S4: Time Management Strategies	Introduce concept of prioritization. Discuss use of lists to improve task completion and breaking tasks into small components to overcome motivation problems. Discuss parent's role in monitoring task completion and planning out tasks (e.g., homework time). Create sample list.
S5: Study Skills	Discuss current test performance and study habits. Introduce active versus passive studying. Complete flashcards and notes from text activities. Create study plan with parent monitoring component. Strengthen commitment to change test scores.
S6: Note Taking	Discuss current practices for retaining material presented in class. Identify benefits of note taking. Provide instruction and feedback on sample notes. Create a contract for note taking during upcoming week with parent monitoring component.
S7: Problem Solving	Discuss goal for problem solving and factors that contribute to problem. Brainstorm solutions and discuss pros and cons of each solution. Outline implementation of selected solution (using contract as needed). Strengthen commitment to plan.

(continued)

TABLE 2.1. *(continued)*

Mobilizing modules	
M1: Engaging the School	Discuss desired level of school staff collaboration. Discuss best ways to communicate with school staff. Strengthen parent motivation to schedule school meeting to discuss home–school collaboration. Review teacher communication strategies.
M2: Habit Formation	Discuss structure of home. Discuss benefit of structure to adolescent and current parent expectations for daily task completion. Create list of morning, school, and evening routine tasks. Discuss monitoring of tasks during next week.
M3: Making an Action Plan	Identify skills and daily tasks that are challenging for adolescent to complete independently. Negotiate home contract for completing these tasks.
M4: Keeping Momentum	Elicit summary of positive changes by family members. Discuss progress on goals. Review use of home contract and family's intention to use STAND tools in future.

Therapists are encouraged to use intuition to design a unique treatment plan for each family. However, in this book, we present sessions in an order that was derived from years of experience delivering STAND. In our own clinic, we have reordered session components several times to find a treatment sequence that seems most palatable and logical. Our current preference for session ordering appears in this book.

It may be useful to repeat modules more than once if a family has not mastered its content. The therapist may choose to do this in a graduated fashion, promoting a family to a new session only after they have fully mastered the current one. It is also possible to return to a session if engagement or skill use wanes over the course of treatment.

Within each module, this book outlines both discussion topics and skills exercises to be performed in session and at home. Therapists are encouraged to elicit family input as they individualize the content of these activities. Individualization of STAND can occur both in choosing session modules and in formulating their precise content. Below is a closer look at how this process of within- and between-session individualization occurs.

Engagement module 1 is designed to introduce treatment as a partnership between the therapist, parent, and teen. The central focus of this module is reviewing available assessment information (see Chapter 3) and asking family members to provide feedback as the therapist articulates case conceptualization. In mapping out each family's unique story, the therapist discusses strengths and priorities, affirming the worth and potential of the parent and teen. This session winds its way into a discussion with the parent about his or her parenting tendencies, the genesis of these patterns, and their influence on the teen. The therapist seeks to leave this session with a clear sense of what deficits the teen is facing, how they impact the teen's life, and how parent behaviors influence these deficits.

In engagement module 2, therapists work with family members to identify and prioritize parent and adolescent areas for change. This process includes identifying the parent's and adolescent's individual treatment goals and selecting modular skills-based components from the treatment menu. Engagement module 3 introduces skills for creating a successful parent–teen partnership—staying calm during stressful discussions, developing listening skills, and communicating honestly and respectfully. The parent and teen plan a meeting at home to practice partnership skills and to discuss their progress on treatment goals. In engagement module 4, the parent and teen discuss ways to create a balance between responsibilities and enjoyable activities at home. This discussion includes a strategy of putting responsibilities before relaxation time and how to make new plans at home through parent–teen collaborative contracting. These contracting skills become an essential part of subsequent skill modules.

For each skill module (1–7), a skill is introduced, a plan for applying the skill is devised, and a parent–teen contract is created to build a contingent home structure that places skill practice before enjoyable activities. The details of skill contracts will vary according to a family's unique home environment and the fun or relaxing activities that a particular teen enjoys.

The mobilizing modules address how to engage the school in treatment, how to turn new skills into habits, and how to create a final action plan that designates the teen's plan for skill practice and how the parent will carry out a home structure that reinforces skill use. Treatment is concluded with a reflection of what has changed and where the family wishes to go next.

Materials

Physical materials required to conduct STAND typically include (1) writing utensils, (2) session worksheets, and (3) adolescent school materials (as applicable). Some modules require additional materials, which are listed at the beginning of each module description. For example, engagement module 2 requires colored pens or markers and index cards to complete the change cards activity (see Chapter 5), and skill module 5 is enhanced if the therapist brings flash cards to session (see Chapter 6).

For organizational purposes, applicable handouts for each module can be found in the pages immediately following module descriptions. However, it is often helpful for therapists to give a bound copy of all worksheets to families during the first session of STAND. Our experience suggests that having a single workbook to bring to therapy each week facilitates family completion of home exercises. Papers are less likely to be lost, and therapists can reference past weeks' content. A workbook also provides families with a handy review of STAND content after treatment ends. To facilitate delivery of materials to families, an ordered set of worksheets can be downloaded and printed (see the box at the end of the Table of Contents).

bound copy to families?

Some activities require the teen to use his or her school materials. Depending on module content, these materials may include a planner or device for recording homework, the student's book bag, binders, folders, study materials, class notes, and homework assignments.

One challenge of working with teens (and sometimes parents) with attention, EF, and motivation difficulties is a tendency to forget materials required for sessions. Our experience suggests that asking families to bring the teen's school materials to every session (regardless of whether they will be utilized) creates an early routine that facilitates readiness for sessions. We typically encourage therapists to provide reminders at the end of sessions if a specific material is necessary to complete the upcoming week's content. However, we do not usually encourage phone calls to remind families to bring materials, as this may stifle the parents' and teens' independent practice of important new skills (i.e., keeping track of required materials).

Sometimes families show up to session without required materials. The therapist then faces a dilemma about whether or not to proceed with the session in light of the missing materials. Treatment setting may dictate whether or not the session should proceed. In our experience, it is usually best to reschedule sessions when materials that are central to the session are forgotten (e.g., the teen forgets to bring his or her backpack to the session on backpack organization). This ensures that content is adequately covered and communicates to families the importance of remembering materials. If repeated forgetfulness interferes with STAND delivery, upfront problem-solving discussions about barriers to preparation or MI aimed at exploring treatment investment may be helpful.

Who Can Deliver STAND?

STAND can be delivered by a range of professionals in a range of settings. Treatment is optimized when the professional has weekly encounters with the parent and teen together for about 1 hour. Professionals who may be well positioned to deliver STAND include psychologists, family counselors, parent advocates, social workers, school psychologists, school counselors, nurses, psychiatrists, coaches, and caseworkers. Delivery settings may include doctor's offices, mental health clinics, private psychology practices, schools, churches, and community centers. We believe that with proper training any invested professional can deliver STAND successfully. In our experience, well-trained individuals with bachelor's degrees can deliver STAND with good fidelity and integrity.

One key to effectively delivering STAND is receiving appropriate exposure to MI prior to treatment delivery. Without these skills, therapists may offer a version of STAND that looks a lot like our first attempt at treating teens with attention, EF, and motivation problems (see Preface)—fraught with parent and teen disengagement and skepticism that can sour families against receiving therapy in the future. We discuss how to develop MI skills in Chapter 4.

Who Is Age Appropriate?

STAND is specifically designed to meet the needs of adolescents. As such, this program assumes that teens are educated in a secondary school environment (with multiple teachers and an expectation of independent academic management). STAND teaches skills that are age appropriate for teens and therefore may be too advanced for elementary-school-age children and too simplistic for adults. STAND also assumes that it is developmentally appropriate for the parent and youth to collaborate; younger children may not be cognitively prepared for this expectation. In spite of the relative immaturity of some adolescents with attention, EF, and motivation problems, our experience and research suggest that STAND is an age-appropriate treatment for adolescents enrolled in middle or high school—typically ages 11–17.

The flexibility of STAND permits treatment to look different for an 11-year-old and a 17-year-old. The key difference in treatment for younger and older adolescents is level of parent scaffolding. Older teens may be able and willing to articulate preferred details of parent–teen contracts. Older youth also may be entrusted with less frequent parental supervision of their skill use. Privileges for older youth should be age appropriate. An 11-year-old may ask for a later bedtime or more screen time (see Bradley in the first example below). A 17-year-old may contract for use of the car or more independence (see Rebecca in the second example below). Following we see how the same session activity may be applied differently for a younger and an older youth.

Bradley

Bradley, a sixth grader, leaned forward in his chair reviewing the contract he and his mother had signed. After some hesitation, he had agreed to write down his homework in a daily agenda in each class. He and his mother had decided that Bradley would be asked to bring the agenda to each teacher after class to obtain a signature for correctly recording his homework assignment. His mother said that she didn't trust him to write it down correctly. She also mentioned that she would send an e-mail to each teacher, explaining the plan. If Bradley didn't go up and get the signature himself, the teacher wasn't going to prompt him. It seemed like a lot to remember. On the other hand, his mother had agreed that for each signature he obtained, he would be allowed to stream one 20-minute episode of his favorite cartoon. She had been so frustrated with him lately that he hadn't been allowed to watch his show in months. He had four teachers, which could mean four episodes each night!

Rebecca

"I don't know about this. I'm not sure I want you snooping in my phone." Rebecca scrolled through the calendar function on her phone. Her high school had recently converted to a "bring your own device" system, allowing students to use tablets and phones to engage in classroom activities. She agreed that she needed to start keeping track of homework better because colleges really care about the junior year. She'd much rather do it on her phone than have to bring some clunky spiral notebook from class to class. Her mother said, "Rebecca, how am I going to make sure that you are doing this if you don't let me see? If you want to use your phone, then I'm going to have to look at it." Rebecca sighed. "Here's the deal," she said. "After school, I'll text you a screenshot of what I've written in each class. As long as I do that, will you promise to let me do my homework at the library with friends instead of coming straight home?" Her mom thought for a minute and then agreed. "I'm willing to try this for 1 week and see where it takes us."

The key for therapists is to assess the teen's readiness for independent skill use. Parents and teens should be engaged in conversations about frequency and type of parent monitoring, age-appropriate responsibility level, and access to enjoyable activities that match the teen's level of independence. The therapist should allow the family to dictate these details, presenting therapy material in a way that encourages flexibility. For example: "For the homework contract, there's a lot of different ways we can set this up depending on the level of independence that you two think Devon is ready to try out."

Who Can Be the Participating Parent?

It is recommended that the primary caretaker participate in treatment with the adolescent. The participating parent must be positioned to monitor the adolescent daily and regulate access to privileges as needed. This means that a parent who lives with the adolescent during the school week typically is best suited for participation in STAND. Correcting maladaptive parenting behaviors that can interfere with teen motivation and skill use is a core element of treatment. Therefore, it is best to engage the parent whose daily behavior has the most influence on the teen's academic habits. Most importantly, the same parent should accompany the teen to treatment each week. Switching off between parents communicates that parent participation in treatment is secondary, disrupts coordination of home activities, and prevents important improvements in parenting behavior.

Sometimes two parents wish to participate in and attend all sessions. This usually works best when both parents share an equal parenting role and have low levels of marital discord. Our experience is that secondary parents often attend a few early sessions and then cease involvement. We always allow both parents to attend session, but treatment is typically easier to deliver when only one parent attends. This allows the focus of activities to remain on the child, avoids marital disagreements that can overtake the session, and prevents two parents from ganging up on a teen. As part of treatment, the primary caretaker can identify strategies for engaging the other parent in new home routines.

Selecting and Prioritizing Treatment Goals

In the spirit of MI, parents and teens are given opportunities to articulate their own treatment goals and choose their own modular treatment components. Families typically know best where problem areas lie and which treatment modules will be most engaging and useful. This client-centered approach does not mean that the therapist must refrain from making suggestions for treatment. After a careful case conceptualization (see Chapter 3), the therapist may have clear ideas about which skill modules will benefit the family most. The therapist can offer these suggestions to the family using the MI framework described in Chapter 4.

Addressing Comorbidities

Teens with attention, EF, and motivation problems often present with comorbidities. These may include anxiety, oppositional behavior, learning disorders, mood problems, or addictive behaviors. The focus of STAND remains attention, EF, and motivation problems; as such, teens whose primary reason for pursuing treatment is outside of these domains should be treated under a different approach or referred to an appropriate specialist. However, when comorbidities are secondary to attention, EF, or motivation problems, STAND may still be appropriate. Some comorbid symptoms may be addressed through the activities in STAND. Others cannot be treated but can be managed to prevent interference with treatment.

Proper assessment and case conceptualization (see Chapter 3) is necessary to determine the hierarchy of an adolescent's presenting problems. When comorbid symptoms are present, the therapist must decide whether modules from another type of treatment should be integrated with STAND or whether treatment of these symptoms should occur separately—either before or after STAND is delivered.

Anxiety

Modest levels of comorbid anxiety symptoms typically do not interfere with STAND delivery. However, STAND does not directly treat anxiety disorders. There is evidence that some youth who present with comorbid anxiety disorders may experience an enhanced response to behavioral treatments for externalizing problems (MTA Cooperative Group, 1999). It is thought that fear of social judgment may motivate these youth to comply highly with treatment activities. To some extent, this appears to be the case in STAND—teens with modest levels of comorbid anxiety are typically more compliant with treatment activities. However, in some cases, extreme anxiety or perfectionism surrounding schoolwork may be a major inhibitor of treatment response, requiring anxiety problems to be treated prior to STAND (see the following example).

Carrie

Sixteen-year-old Carrie was referred to treatment by her mother for problems with time management during schoolwork. Carrie's mother reported that she had been diagnosed with ADHD in early elementary school and had a history of completing schoolwork very slowly. Carrie's mother reported that as an 11th grader Carrie typically works on homework until 2:00 or 3:00 in the morning, preventing her from obtaining adequate sleep. Carrie's mother reported frequent arguments with Carrie related to her bedtime. Carrie reported that she felt unable to go to sleep until her schoolwork was complete.

During treatment, it became increasingly clear that Carrie's time management problems stemmed less from slow mental processing or difficulties with EF and more from an intense fear of turning in imperfect work. Carrie refused to move on to a new assignment until she had repeatedly checked and rechecked her work. After a careful discussion with Carrie and her mother, treatment shifted focus to cognitive-behavioral therapy aimed at reducing Carrie's perfectionistic approach to schoolwork. The therapist and family agreed to reevaluate whether components of STAND were appropriate once Carrie's anxiety was managed.

Depression

If depression is a primary presenting concern, the teen should participate in an appropriate therapy to address these symptoms prior to beginning STAND components. However, some teens whose primary concern is EF or motivation problems may present with modest depressive symptoms. If depression is conceptualized as a reaction to academic or family stressors stemming from attention, EF, or motivation problems, improving functioning in these domains may alleviate symptoms of depression. In addition, behavioral activation associated with completion of weekly STAND activities may serve to reduce depressive symptoms. Therapists are encouraged to conduct proper risk assessment procedures should depressive symptoms persist or worsen during treatment.

Oppositional Behavior

Oppositional behavior is among the most common comorbid presenting problems for teens with attention deficits. Highly oppositional teens may threaten the safety or stability of a household. Some parents cannot engage the teen in collaboration, which may mean an inability to bring the teen to session, difficulty locating the teen, or aggressive behavior toward family members when they attempt to place limits on the teen. In these cases of extreme oppositional behavior, the family may require intensive services aimed at helping the parent regain control of the teen's behavior.

Although oppositional behavior is a common comorbidity for teens with attention, EF, and motivation problems, most teens who completed STAND in our clinic were cooperative and respectful to therapists and parents during session. We believe this has much to do with the person-centered MI perspective from which STAND is delivered.

Some oppositional behaviors may be addressed in STAND without adjunctive efforts. For example, teens with moderate levels of anger or defiance may make disrespectful comments to parents who restrict access to enjoyable activities or may argue when parents ask them to begin homework. Parent–teen communication skills introduced in treatment can be emphasized at home as a part of treatment. If needed, contracts can stipulate the number of disrespectful comments a teen may display during homework time before enjoyable activities can no longer be accessed. Data from our pilot study demonstrate that oppositional behavior decreases substantially during treatment. This may largely occur as a function of an improved parent–teen relationship that reduces coercive interactions.

Oppositional behavior can also be effectively managed during sessions. The MI approach naturally reduces in-session oppositional behavior by respecting a teen's voice and avoiding didactic and contentious interactions between the therapist and the teen. During sessions, some parents even adopt the interaction style modeled by the therapist, which naturally reduces conflict. In Chapter 8 we outline a range of additional strategies for effectively managing high levels of oppositional behavior and parent–teen conflict in session.

How Much Change Is Expected?

Neurocognitive deficits associated with attention, EF, and motivation problems are typically chronic—meaning that full remission of symptoms is not expected. Progress for teens who struggle in these areas is typically slow and unfolds over many years. STAND aims to lay the groundwork for steady improvement in attention, EF, and motivation domains by teaching compensatory skills, helping teens and parents to set clear and meaningful goals for the future, and forging realistic plans for maintaining adaptive parent and teen habits.

During STAND, many adolescents show stark initial improvements in attention, EF skills, or motivation when the program is new, contingent home structure is first implemented, and desire to please the therapist is high. In some cases, this initial progress is maintained across therapy. In other cases, initial progress declines midway through therapy, possibly due to parental failure to consistently monitor and reinforce skill practice or to lost interest in participation. It is our experience that progress will return once the issues that led to a decline in skill use are exposed, discussed, and resolved with the family. Allowing these issues to be addressed in therapy promotes family awareness of inconsistent teen or parent strategy use. Advice for addressing slow or inconsistent progress is found in Chapter 8.

Booster Sessions to Maintain Change

In our randomized controlled trial of STAND, improvements in adolescent functioning were maintained 6 months after treatment. However, parent reinforcement of a consistent home structure decreased somewhat. It may be the case that parents no longer implement short-term behavior management strategies because teens are independently managing their academics. However, parents and teens also may continue to struggle with long-term motivation and maintaining a consistent routine that emphasizes accountability.

In the final mobilizing module, families discuss plans for relapse prevention—and what to do if functioning slides. Sometimes major life changes can trigger new problems; other times families slowly stop practicing a previously successful home routine. Families should be encouraged to recontact the therapist in the future should progress slow or reverse.

Therapists who conduct booster sessions with a family can systematically assess the family's reason for returning to treatment and can select STAND components that appear best suited to address the family's residual difficulties.

Delivering Treatment in a Group

In certain settings, there may be benefits to delivering STAND in a group rather than in a dyad. Groups may be more cost-effective or may allow treatment of more families when clinician time is limited. Group-delivered treatment also allows parents and teens to benefit from social support and shared experiences with similar others and can increase the credibility of intervention skills.

When STAND is delivered in a group, treatment is less individualized, families do not receive as much personalized MI, and less attention is available to address family-specific treatment issues, such as failure to complete home exercises and nonresponse to home contracts. In general, therapist-conducted MI discussions are replaced by group conversations.

The recommended format for delivering STAND as a group is a mix of parent-only, teen-only, and parent–teen collaborative group activities. Whereas individual sessions are designed to be an hour, we find that 90 minutes is necessary for group sessions in order to account for late arrivals, room changes, and questions. Following is an example of a schedule for a group session:

00:00–00:15—Parent–teen collaborative homework review

00:15–01:15—Skill introduction (parent and teen groups meet alone)

01:15–01:30—Collaborative parent–teen group activity and home activity

Using this format, two rooms are necessary to accommodate separate parent and teen groups. The two groups start together in one room, and either the parent or the teen group breaks out to a separate room for the skill introduction parts of the session. Additionally, two therapists are needed to separately run simultaneous parent and teen groups.

Our experience is that a community-based parent training model (Cunningham, 2006) works well for delivery of STAND in separate parent and teen groups. This model uses a facilitative problem-solving approach. In this model, parents or teens sit at separate tables of four to six individuals and form subgroups. A subgroup leader is elected to take notes on subgroup proceedings and report back to the larger group. Subgroups hold time-limited discussions on topics prompted by the therapist. After subgroup discussions, the therapist facilitates large-group discussion of points summarized by subgroup leaders.

Adolescent groups are best organized with considerations for age. Typically, separating older and younger adolescents best serves the therapeutic process. Behavior management in session may be necessary, particularly for younger teens. For example, a raffle ticket system can be used to promote participation and rule following. For each 15-minute interval of good participation and respectful behavior, teens can be issued a raffle ticket. At the end of the full program, staff can hold a raffle for developmentally appropriate prizes (e.g., music downloads, coffee gift cards, gift certificates to popular restaurants).

Group content can generally follow session content presented in Chapters 5–7. MI can be replaced with subgroup discussions. The therapist can practice MI when responding to parent comments in a large group. (For more information on delivering MI in groups, see Wagner & Ingersoll, 2013). Throughout Chapters 5–7, session content that is particularly well suited to group parent–teen collaborative activity is indicated with a ✪. I provide a sample curriculum for conducting STAND as an 8-week group in Table 2.2.

Therapists are encouraged to outline a STAND group curriculum prior to beginning a group cycle. Key considerations are the number of sessions, length of sessions, content of sessions, and behavior management system for teens.

This Book

The remaining chapters in this book discuss how to translate a strong case conceptualization into an individualized treatment plan (Chapter 3), blend MI into skills-based treatment (Chapter 4), and outline the content of each STAND module (Chapters 5–7). I close by offering clinical advice on a range of difficult issues that our team has observed during treatment (Chapter 8). My goal is to provide a meaningful reference for professionals in a variety of settings who work with families of adolescents who struggle with attention, EF, and motivation problems.

TABLE 2.2. Delivering STAND in a Group

	Parent content	Teen content	Collaborative in-session activity	Collaborative home activity
Session 1	• Discuss attention, EF, and motivation problems. • How do problems affect family and school? • Discuss common parenting patterns.	• Discuss attention, EF, and motivation problems. • How do problems affect family and school? • Discuss your strengths.	Parent–teen discussion of parent and teen strengths and how attention, EF, and motivation problems influence academics and family functioning.	Into the Future
Session 2	• Change card activity • Set three personal goals for treatment.	• Change card activity. • Set three personal goals for treatment.	Parent–teen comparison of change cards, prioritization of change cards, and discussion of goals.	Letter from the Future activity
Session 3	• Reflective listening • "I" statements • Home Privilege Inventory	• Reflective listening • "I" statements • Home Privilege Inventory	Negotiate home contract for completion of a daily chore.	Implement home contract for completion of a daily chore.
Session 4	• Discuss how teens keep track of homework. • Discuss book bag organization.	• Discuss keeping track of homework. • Reorganize book bag with peers.	Negotiate home contract for either recording homework or book bag organization.	Implement home contract.
Session 5	• Discuss monitoring homework and study skills. • Introduce homework to-do list and active study skills.	• Introduce homework to-do list. • Introduce Active Study Skills.	Negotiate homework contract.	Implement homework contract. Use either active study skills or homework to-do list at least once.
Session 6	• List daily routine tasks for adolescent. • Discuss benefits of routine.	• List daily routine tasks for adolescent. • Discuss benefits of routine.	Parent and teen compare daily routine tasks and create a list of tasks to track for 1 week.	Parent and teen separately track completion of all tasks on list for 1 week.

(continued)

TABLE 2.2. (continued)

	Parent content	Teen content	Collaborative in-session activity	Collaborative home activity
Session 7	• Select tasks from daily routine that were difficult for teen to complete. • Discuss effective versus ineffective privileges.	• Select tasks from daily routine that were difficult for teen to complete. • Discuss desired privileges.	Negotiate full home contract based on agreed-upon tasks from the task list and privileges.	Implement full home contract.
Session 8	• Discuss ways school may support teen skill use. • Discuss appropriate home–school collaboration. • Discuss strategies for engaging teachers.	• Discuss strategies for retaining lectures. • Note-taking training • Discuss strategies for building positive teacher relationships.	Discuss level of communication that is needed between parent, teen, and teacher.	Identify point person at school to facilitate communication.

CHAPTER 3

Case Conceptualization

Family-Informed Case Conceptualization

The difficulties of adolescents with attention, EF, and motivation problems vary widely. Thus, from a behavioral perspective, careful assessment is needed to focus the nature and goals of treatment—especially for a program with individualized components. When a therapist possesses keen understanding of the unique deficits and impairments of an adolescent, the youth is served with optimally tailored care. Given the parent–teen collaborative nature of STAND, thorough case conceptualization also includes assessment of parent behavior and parent–teen interaction styles.

Case conceptualization in STAND is viewed as a collaborative effort between the parent, teen, and therapist. The goal of case conceptualization in STAND is mutual understanding of treatment's focus. Together, the therapist and the family members identify behaviors that might be changed during treatment to meet each individual's goals.

To conceptualize a case, information about the family must be collected, reviewed with the parent and teen, and collaboratively interpreted. For efficiency, it is recommended that information gathering begin prior to the start of treatment through records collection and an assessment session attended by the parent and the teen. Starting assessment prior to treatment will prepare the therapist to begin case conceptualization with family members in engagement module 1 (see Chapter 5). Before engagement module 2, the therapist is encouraged to review the working case conceptualization and to use this formulation to create change cards (see engagement module 2; Chapter 5) that identify key targets for parent and adolescent change.

Assessment Philosophy: Consideration of Both Strengths and Difficulties

Understanding and affirming the strengths and worth of families is an important component of change-focused therapy. Frequent discussion of strengths, interests, and values creates neutrality in session that prevents demoralization caused by over-emphasis on difficulties. Treatment that emphasizes strengths necessitates assessment that includes strength-based inventories. When a therapist integrates teens' and parents' positive qualities into the case conceptualization, the therapist also prepares for a compassionate approach to treatment that acknowledges client worth.

Sources of Information

The assessment process involves collecting information from a variety of sources and conceptualizing difficulties across a variety of domains. The daily environment of teens with attention, EF, and motivation problems presents endemic challenges to accurate assessment of teen functioning. For this reason, a multisource approach to assessment is critical. Sometimes multisource assessment leads to contradictory accounts of teen or parent behavior. It is the therapist's job to disentangle these discrepancies collaboratively with the family. Inconsistencies may indicate behavior that varies by setting, the presence of informant perceptual biases, or a reporter with insufficient information to offer an accurate report.

There are specific challenges to assessment in this population. Teens with attention, EF, and motivation problems may underreport their difficulties because they are unaware of their deficits, embarrassed by their difficulties, or just impatient or inattentive during the assessment process. Parents may be excellent reporters about home behavior but may know less about academic and behavioral functioning that occurs at school or in the presence of peers. Some parents may possess overly negative views of the adolescent caused by years of negative interactions. These beliefs can cloud the parent's objectivity. Obtaining reports from the adolescent's teachers may be beneficial to the assessment of school functioning, but secondary school teacher reports are often challenging to obtain. Some teachers are only vaguely acquainted with students because of the impersonal nature of many secondary school settings.

In the face of these assessment challenges, the clinician is charged with cobbling together an accurate assessment of the teen's functioning. Our general recommendation is to obtain information from as many sources as possible across relevant domains. Parents and adolescents should be engaged foremost. Teacher ratings should be kept brief and can be channeled toward a teacher who knows the adolescent best or in whose class the adolescent struggles most. Reaching secondary school teachers via e-mail appears to work well. Direct observation of adolescent skills (e.g., looking at the teen's backpack or daily planner, observations during assessment) and official records (e.g., school grades, disciplinary records) can provide objective supplements to subjective teen, parent, and teacher reports.

Recommended Measures

There is a range of measures that can be used to assess each domain of functioning (see Table 3.1 on the next page).

A pretreatment interview with the parent and/or teen can aid in understanding an adolescent's history and present functioning. A unique benefit of interviewing the family members is the ability to obtain qualitative information about adolescent and parent strengths and difficulties. In addition, an interview format allows the therapist to ask follow-up questions or employ a functional analytic approach to ask about typical antecedents to behaviors (what typically triggers or leads up to the problem), the details of the behavior (what usually happens), and the natural consequences of the behavior (what happens after the behavior occurs).

In Figure 3.1 on page 37 we offer sample questions for a semistructured clinical interview with the parent. ⟶ AAPC & PAMS

Rating scales can be a time-saving approach to collecting systematic information from families about specific problem areas or symptom clusters. Domains that are successfully assessed via rating scale and specific recommended measures are listed in Table 3.1. Two rating scales that were developed and validated by our team for use when delivering STAND—the Adolescent Academic Problems Checklist (AAPC; Sibley, Altszuler, Morrow, & Merrill, 2014) and the Parent Academic Management Scale (PAMS; Sibley et al., 2016)—are provided at the end of this chapter. The AAPC is a clinician-friendly measure that can be administered to parents, teens, or teachers and that assesses the extent to which adolescents use compensatory organization skills to manage daily academics. The PAMS assesses parent academic involvement specific to the management of teen organization, time management, and planning. The information on the PAMS can be used to detect whether the parent displays a collaborative, uninvolved, or controlling academic involvement pattern.

Grade book data can be obtained from a school's online grade book to provide a detailed record of the adolescent's academic performance. Across classes, the therapist can view the adolescent's assignment completion rate, performance on tests and quizzes, and performance on completed assignments. The therapist can compare homework grades with classwork grades and view differences between performance on short-term and long-term assignments. Through analysis of these records, the therapist is well positioned to detect patterns in the teen's academic functioning that may indicate optimal intervention targets.

Many psychometricians assess teen deficits through cognitive tasks that directly measure abilities across a broad spectrum of cognitive functions. Although these assessments can provide interesting information about a teen's underlying *abilities*,

TABLE 3.1. Suggested Methods of Assessment for Case Conceptualization

	Teen	Parent	Teacher	Records	Observation
Teen Functioning					
Psychosocial history	Interview	Interview	—	Past grades	—
Strengths and values	Interview	Interview	Written list	Current grades	In-session behavior
Academics	Interview	Interview	—	Current grades	—
Home behavior	Interview	Interview	—	—	—
Parent–teen relationship	Conflict Behavior Questionnaire[a]	Conflict Behavior Questionnaire[a]	—	—	In-session behavior
Teen deficits					
Executive functioning skills	Adolescent Academic Problems Checklist[b]	Adolescent Academic Problems Checklist[b]	Adolescent Academic Problems Checklist[b]	—	Book bag organization and planner use
Motivation	Quick Delay Questionnaire[c]	Quick Delay Questionnaire[c]	—	—	—
Attention	ADHD Symptom Checklist	ADHD Symptom Checklist	ADHD Symptom Checklist	—	In-session behavior
Parent					
Strengths and values	Interview	Interview	—	—	In-session behavior
Academic Involvement		Parent Academic Management Scale[b]			In session behavior
Stress	—	Caregiver Strain Questionnaire[d]	—	—	—

[a]Robin and Foster (1995); [b]included at the end of this chapter; [c]Clare, Helps, and Sonuga-Barke (2010); [d]Brannan, Heflinger, and Bickman (1997).

- Why are you currently seeking treatment?
- Describe the teen's (organization skills, homework skills, test performance, time management, work quality, behavior at home/school).
- In what ways is the teen motivated to do schoolwork or household chores? In what ways does he or she struggle with motivation?
- What is your role (parent) in supporting or managing the teen's academics and daily routine?
- When did you first notice problems in school/at home?
- Has the teen received any clinical diagnoses? If so, when and by whom?
- Were there any notable stressors or health events in the teen's life that we should know about?
- What stressors does the teen face today?
- Who lives in the home?
- What are the interactions like between the teen and each family member?
- What responsibilities does the teen have at home?
- Where does the teen go to school? What is his or her educational placement? Does he or she have an IEP or 504 plan?
- When he or she was younger, what was the teen's class placement? When did he or she receive an IEP?
- What are the teen's current and previous grades in school (by year)?
- Has the teen ever been suspended or disciplined by the school? If so, for what type of incident?
- Has the teen ever received educational testing (such as an IQ or diagnostic test)?
- Who administered this testing and when was it done?
- How frequently do you communicate with the teen's school? What was your communication with the school like when the teen was younger?
- Has the teen participated in any past treatment for school or behavioral difficulties?
- Has the teen ever taken medication for these difficulties? If so, what type and dose?
- How has your approach to parenting the teen changed as he or she has gotten older?

FIGURE 3.1. Sample interview questions for parent or teen interview.

they can be expensive and lengthy to administer and do not offer information about a teen's *performance* in daily life. Cognitive tasks do not offer information about compensatory skills that the teen utilizes to overcome deficits. Not only do these tasks fail to account for compensatory abilities, but they are also sensitive to situational influences that may affect task performance on a given day. As a result, they are most useful when interpreted in conjunction with information about a teen's daily functioning.

Case Impressions

Prior to engagement module 1, the therapist can gather and score all information collected in the preceding assessment session. During engagement module 1, information collected in each domain of functioning listed in Table 3.1 can be briefly reviewed with family members. Family members offer their impressions of the therapist's interpretation, collaboratively refining case conceptualization in session.

Details:

- *Parent reports 20 hours of academic involvement per week.*
- *PAMS: reports daily monitoring of online grade book and daily checking of homework.*
- *PAMS: reports doing homework for the adolescent weekly.*
- *PAMS: reports no use of rewards, privileges, or contracts to reinforce success.*
- *Parent Interview: complained that she must sit down and hover over adolescent to get him to start homework, creates a lot of arguments.*
- *Adolescent Interview: teen explained that he liked his mother's help because it made homework easier.*
- *Observation: adolescent's book bag was very clean, mother reported that she organizes it with him every Sunday night.*

Impressions:

- *PAMS: reports daily monitoring of online grade book and daily checking of homework. Mother appears heavily involved in academics to the point of inappropriately doing some tasks for the teen. Teen may be unmotivated to complete work independently knowing his mother will eventually help. Accountability appears low (no use of contingencies).*

FIGURE 3.2. Summary of parent academic involvement.

The therapist can prepare for engagement module 1 by organizing information collected in the assessment session by domain. This process includes carefully reviewing all materials and summarizing points across sources and measures (for an example, see Figure 3.2).

This process can be completed for each domain, allowing the therapist to organize impressions prior to engagement module 1.

Presenting Case Impressions in Engagement Module I

One of the aims of engagement module 1 is to provide family members with feedback on information gathered during the assessment session. With the notes taken prior to the session, the therapist systematically reviews information collected in each domain. Discussion of case impressions follows the elicit–provide–elicit approach (EPE) described in Miller and Rollnick (2013) and introduced in Chapter 4. Using the EPE approach, the therapist begins by *eliciting* the parent's and teen's knowledge about a certain domain. Following the family's answer, the therapist asks permission to *provide* feedback on the family's functioning in the domain. Finally, the therapist asks the family members to share their reaction to the information given by the therapist. A key consideration when practicing EPE is to keep therapist's comments relatively brief, allowing the family members to do most of the talking. In addition, because assessment feedback involves discussion of the teen's areas of difficulty, it is important for the therapist to regularly affirm the teen's (and parent's) worth and strengths, communicating empathy during the interaction. The therapist can introduce the discussion by asking the family's permission to discuss the topic (see engagement module 1 for example dialogue). Once the therapist repeats this process for each domain, a summary can be provided to the family that integrates information provided by the therapist with the family member's feedback. At the end of the summary, the therapist should consult the family about its accuracy (see Chapter 4).

Further description of EPE, affirming clients, providing summaries, and other relevant aspects of MI during this phase of treatment can be found in Chapter 4. Chapter 5 contains a detailed overview of the content of engagement module 1, including all components relevant to delivering case impressions.

Finalizing Case Conceptualization

Following engagement module 1, the therapist is equipped with initial case impressions, family feedback on these impressions, and summary of the case that was presented to and affirmed by the parent and the teen. It may be useful to provide a written narrative summary of each family member's strengths, areas of impairment, and factors that contribute to impairments (see Figures 3.3 and 3.4 on pages 40 and 41). The working case conceptualization can guide the therapist's selection of change cards (discussed next) to bring to engagement module 2.

Creating Change Cards

3-4 cards in e.1. module

Change cards are a set of index cards each of which identifies one key area for change articulated by the parent and teen in engagement module 1. Based on the case conceptualization discussion in engagement module 1, the therapist can prepare change cards for the family to review in engagement module 2. The therapist should aim to create an equal number of change cards for the parent and for the teen— typically three or four cards per participant. Doing so communicates their mutual participation in treatment.

Change cards should be worded positively to represent possibilities for the future rather than parent or adolescent weaknesses. They should directly represent areas for change articulated by parents and teens in engagement module 1 rather than the therapist's opinions. However, deliberately wording change cards is a strategy that can facilitate appropriate treatment focusing. We can consider the cases of Arthur and Amber in devising sample change cards for engagement module 2.

Arthur

Based on the case conceptualization, key problem areas articulated for Arthur include missing homework assignments, needing reminders to get started on work, failing to keep track of assignments, and experiencing motivation problems during homework or other boring tasks (such as chores). Key problem areas articulated by Arthur's

Name: *Arthur K.*

Age: *14*

Grade: *8*

School Setting: *Regular + Resource Room*

Medication Status: *Concerta 54 mg, once daily on weekdays*

Parent Relationship to Teen: *Biological Mother*

Overview and History: *Arthur is an Asian American male who lives with his mother, a single parent, who works full-time as a dental hygienist. A testing report and Individualized Education Plan (IEP) provided by Arthur's mother indicate that he possesses above-average intelligence and was in regular classes at his local public school up until the fifth grade. In sixth grade, Arthur began to experience homework problems and qualified for an IEP under the Other Health Impaired category following a diagnosis of attention-deficit/hyperactivity disorder by his pediatrician. His mother reports being unsure of this diagnosis, mentioning that he became lazy at the transition to middle school and seems to lack passion for anything besides video games. His mother reports no involvement in academics, aside from attending annual IEP meetings and parent–teacher conferences as requested by the school. She reports that the medication helps Arthur remain focused and that Arthur complains about taking his pill but is very compliant with her request that he do so daily.*

Strengths and Values: *Arthur is involved in swim team and has been competing regionally since he was 8. He enjoys taking apart electronics and playing video games. His mother reports that he always follows rules, and his teacher reported that he is respectful to adults and classmates. Arthur reported that school is important to him but wasn't sure why. His mother reported that she also values education and helping Arthur to develop successful interests. She also stated that her parenting strengths include always finding time to spend with her son, despite being a single parent who works full time. She said she and Arthur rarely argue.*

Teen Functioning: *Arthur currently receives B's and C's in his classes. According to his online grade book, his test grades are typically in the A range. He misses about 20% of his homework assignments, particularly in math class, where this number is closer to 40%. At home, Arthur is expected to do several chores that include washing dishes after dinner and taking out the trash once a week. He performs these chores without complaints, but his mother reports that she must remind him to do so.*

Parenting: *Arthur's mother does not report any daily academic involvement, aside from insisting that he sit down to begin homework immediately after swim practice. She reports low conflict with her son. Her primary strategy for supporting his deficits is providing reminders.*

Contributing Factors: *With respect to his missing assignments, Arthur and his mother reported high motivation problems on the Quick Delay Questionnaire, which may indicate a tendency to avoid mentally effortful assignments. Arthur's teacher and mother report no use of compensatory skills to keep track of homework or store his completed homework in an organized manner. His mother does not provide accountability at home for homework tracking or completion. She expresses beliefs that she is too busy to help and that he is old enough to manage work on his own.*

FIGURE 3.3. Working case conceptualization for Arthur.

Name: Amber P.

Age: 16

Grade: 10

School Setting: Regular

Medication Status: None

Parent Relationship to Teen: Biological Mother

Overview and History: Amber is a European American female who resides with her mother (a stay-at-home mom), father (a police captain), and older brother. Amber attends private Catholic school and possesses a Section 504 plan at school that allows her to take extra time on tests, preferential classroom seating, and testing in a quiet environment. Amber has attended the same Catholic school since she was in prekindergarten. Her mother reports she has always struggled with test taking, completing homework in a timely manner, and participating in the classroom. She has received accommodations through her 504 plan since second grade. She has always made C's and D's in her classes, with occasional F's. Every summer since seventh grade, she's had to repeat at least one class during summer school (the subjects have varied).

Strengths and Values: Amber is reported to be very social, possessing many friends at school and is a star player on her high school volleyball team. She enjoys sports and traveling abroad with her cousins during summer vacation. Her mother describes her as very caring, and Amber states that her family is important to her. As a parent, Amber's mom says that she is the first to volunteer at the school, that she is willing to do anything to give Amber the resources she needs to succeed (including spending a lot of money on tutors and learning programs), and that she feels that she and her daughter possess a close relationship, despite the fact that she believes that Amber has a bad attitude when asked to complete work or chores. Amber's mother values education and hopes her daughter will be able to play volleyball in college.

Teen Functioning: Amber's low grades in school appear mostly caused by poor test grades. Her work completion was relatively high (very few missing assignments). Her teacher and mother report that she fails to study for tests and quizzes unless a tutor guides studying. Without the tutor, she moves very slowly through homework assignments, often going to bed after midnight. The teacher reports that homework assignments are turned in but not completed thoroughly because Amber tends to make careless mistakes on her assignments.

Parenting: Amber's mother reports a history of high involvement in homework but recently began relying on a tutor to ensure work completion. She frequently removes Amber's access to her cell phone for weeks when she receives poor test grades. She reports that she lectures Amber when she doesn't study for tests, stating a belief that Amber does not seem to understand the link between hard work and success in school.

Contributing Factors: Amber's poor test performance may stem from a combination of factors that include insufficient time spent studying, failure to take notes in class, and reliance on a tutor to create study guides, cheating herself of important interaction with test material. Amber may struggle with motivation during study time, as well as insufficient EF skills related to coordinating study for a test. Her mother's long-term removal of a privilege that could be highly motivating may be preventing effective daily contingency management.

FIGURE 3.4. Working case conceptualization for Amber.

mother include an overreliance on providing reminders and not having enough time to help her son with schoolwork. Another implicit problem was Arthur's mother's belief that parents should not be involved in teen academics. These problem areas can become positively worded areas for change that directly link to parent and teen discussions in engagement module 1 (see Figure 3.5).

With respect to the final change card in Figure 3.5, a parent may possess a maladaptive belief that she or he should not be involved in any aspect of adolescent academics. Many times, this belief is mitigated in engagement module 1 (see Chapter 5) through an MI-framed discussion of typical parenting patterns among parents of teens with attention, EF, and motivation problems. One way of ensuring that the parent feels her or his belief is heard and respected, without reinforcing its maladaptive nature, is to provide a change card that is an agreeable reframing. In this case, the belief that a parent should not be involved in academics can be reflected in the text "create structure that requires independence." The change card is anchored in the parent's articulated value and goal for teen independence. The reframing is an addition to the card about creating structure. Here the therapist emphasizes the

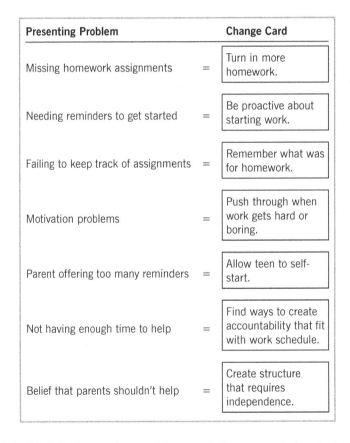

Presenting Problem		Change Card
Missing homework assignments	=	Turn in more homework.
Needing reminders to get started	=	Be proactive about starting work.
Failing to keep track of assignments	=	Remember what was for homework.
Motivation problems	=	Push through when work gets hard or boring.
Parent offering too many reminders	=	Allow teen to self-start.
Not having enough time to help	=	Find ways to create accountability that fit with work schedule.
Belief that parents shouldn't help	=	Create structure that requires independence.

FIGURE 3.5. Presenting problems and change cards for Arthur.

parent's role in promoting independence, which was an important parent value, while framing independence as a consequence of parent actions. Through the process of obtaining family feedback on change cards, the therapist allows the parent to reject or modify the card if he or she does not relate to its content (see Chapter 5).

Amber

Based on the case conceptualization discussion, key problem areas articulated for Amber included insufficient time spent studying for tests, relying on a tutor to direct studying, disengagement during class, and not completing work thoroughly. The only key problem area articulated by Amber's mom was an overreliance on lecturing and privilege removal to discipline Amber for her poor grades. In this case, more problems are articulated for the teen than the parent, requiring the therapist to contrive a balanced set of change cards. The therapist picks up on the mixed consequences of using a tutor. This dilemma is converted to a change card that is presented to the family. The sample list of change cards for Amber and her mom are offered in Figure 3.6.

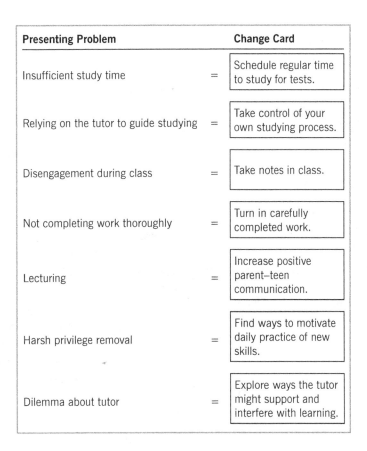

Presenting Problem		Change Card
Insufficient study time	=	Schedule regular time to study for tests.
Relying on the tutor to guide studying	=	Take control of your own studying process.
Disengagement during class	=	Take notes in class.
Not completing work thoroughly	=	Turn in carefully completed work.
Lecturing	=	Increase positive parent–teen communication.
Harsh privilege removal	=	Find ways to motivate daily practice of new skills.
Dilemma about tutor	=	Explore ways the tutor might support and interfere with learning.

FIGURE 3.6. Presenting problems and change cards for Amber.

Change cards operate much like a therapeutic reflection (see Chapter 4) in MI. They are guesses at what the parent or the teen meant when he or she was describing problems at home. Some change cards reflect explicit utterances by the parent or teen. Others may reflect implicit concerns that were not articulated but were sensed by the therapist. All change cards above reflect content derived from the parent's or adolescent's stories, rather than judgments from the therapist. In presenting change cards to the parent and teen, the therapist invites family feedback on the list to ensure that it accurately captures areas of change that feel relevant to families. Figure 3.7 lists sample change card wordings that have been popular in our clinic.

Sample Teen Change Cards	Sample Parent Change Cards
• Develop a positive relationship with teachers. • Earn access to more activities with friends. • Finish homework earlier. • Spend more time studying. • Increase test scores. • Improve study skills. • Manage time better after school. • Make good decisions about how to spend your time. • Feel prepared for tests. • Keep belongings organized. • Learn to shift gears and stop working. • Plan ahead for long-term projects. • Complete more homework assignments. • Become comfortable asking teacher for accommodations. • Turn in schoolwork on time. • Stay on task during homework time. • Learn to ignore distractions. • Develop a system for keeping track of homework. • Write in daily planner during each class. • Start homework without being reminded. • Complete morning routine independently.	• Find more time for yourself. • Create clear structure at home. • Build teen motivation to complete assignments. • Implement consequences more consistently. • Reduce homework helping. • Help teen find ways to get started on assignments. • Give teen opportunities to prove his or her independence. • Find out what motivates teen. • Allow teen to independently prioritize assignments. • Reduce anxiety about adolescent failure. • Give teen a chance to work independently before helping. • Find ways to hold teen accountable for work. • Monitor schoolwork more often. • Find a balance with assistance and independence. • Pay more attention to self-care. • Follow through on delivering rewards. • Organize own weekly schedule. • Feel more comfortable backing off of school help. • Use privileges to motivate work completion. • Stay calmer when delivering consequences. • Effectively communicate with teachers. • Acknowledge teen's small successes. • Reduce reminders.

FIGURE 3.7. Sample wording of teen and parent change card.

Using Case Conceptualization to Focus Treatment

In engagement module 2 (see Chapter 5), the therapist can present the change cards to the family, obtain family feedback on the relevance and wording of each card, and encourage parents and teens to remove or add cards based on their personal preferences. Once the pruning of cards is complete, family members can be asked to collaboratively prioritize cards in order of perceived urgency.

As the parent and teen make clear their individual priorities for treatment, the therapist guides each family member to convert change cards into personal treatment goals. The parent and teen each choose three goals related to personal changes they would like to see themselves make during STAND. With change cards and goals laid out on the table, the therapist can then turn toward the treatment menu (see Chapter 5) and guide the parent and teen to select individualized skill modules that support their priorities. *change cards → tx goals → tx "menu" for skills*

In sum, the primary purpose of case conceptualization is appropriate focusing of treatment to target domains that are both relevant and meaningful to each individual family member. As a secondary benefit, the therapist gains a careful understanding of the family that will increase the sensitivity with which treatment is delivered. We have seen how case conceptualization begins with collection of information from

---

Seven change cards were presented to Amber and her mother. Amber agreed that the cards seemed appropriate but stated that she was not interested in taking notes in class because no one else did and the teacher gave PowerPoint presentations. Amber's mom remarked that she thought note taking would help her tremendously to retain material. Amber agreed to keep it on the list because her mother liked it but said she would make no promises about taking notes. Amber's mother agreed with all cards and commented that she had recently been ambivalent about the tutor and thought it would be a good idea to discuss what role might be appropriate. Amber and her mother collaboratively prioritized the change cards in the following order: Take control of your own studying process, Find ways to motivate daily practice of new skills, Schedule regular time to study for tests, Turn in carefully completed work, Increase positive parent–teen communication, Take notes in class, and Explore ways the tutor might support and interfere with learning. Amber's three therapy goals included getting her mom to trust her so she doesn't have to receive so many lectures, bringing her test average up to a C, and not failing any classes this year. Mom's goals included staying patient when Amber brings home a poor grade, finding motivators for Amber, and being more consistent with her rules at home. Based on the discussions in session, Amber and her mom selected from the treatment menu the following skill modules: preparing for tests, note taking, and making a homework plan.

FIGURE 3.8. Therapist contact note for Amber.

multiple sources and measures and how careful therapist analysis of materials builds a story that connects deficits and environmental factors with the challenges of daily life. We have seen how the therapist can take this story to the family and ask for feedback, listening to and reflecting aspects of the narrative that seem most urgent or important to the parent and teen. Finally, the therapist is able to capture these priorities and articulate them to family members in wording that promotes positive change, leading family members to focus their own goals for treatment.

Figure 3.8 on the previous page contains a therapist contact note summarizing how this process concluded for Amber's family.

RATING SCALE 3.1. Adolescent Academic Problems Checklist (AAPC)

To be completed by parent, teacher, or teen. Please describe the adolescent.	Not at all	Just a little	Pretty much	Very much
1. Fails to take class notes				
2. Receives poor grades on tests/quizzes				
3. Does not follow through on homework instructions				
4. Is disruptive in class				
5. Does not follow through on instructions given during class				
6. Arrives late for class				
7. Does not study for tests/quizzes				
8. Turns in work that was not completed thoroughly				
9. Has poorly organized folders or binders				
10. Forgets to bring appropriate materials to class				
11. Fails to turn in homework that he or she has already completed				
12. Fails to turn in assignments on time				
13. Actively refuses to complete work				
14. Has difficulty organizing writing assignments				
15. Is noncompliant with adult requests				
16. Makes careless errors on work				
17. Fails to record homework assignments in a daily planner				
18. Fails to participate in class discussions				
19. Is off task during schoolwork				
20. Fails to raise hand before speaking in class				
21. Leaves longer-term projects until the last minute				
22. Skips class for unexcused reasons				
23. Poor time management				
24. Has difficulty getting started on assignments				

(continued)

Scoring and Interpretation

The AAPC can be interpreted by examining individual items for clinical elevations (*pretty much* or *very much*) that may indicate key targets for treatment.

Severity indices can also be computed for:

Academic Executive Functioning Skills. The following items can be averaged to provide a severity index (ranging from 0 = *not at all* to 3 = *very much*): 1, 2, 3, 5, 7, 8, 9, 10, 11, 12, 14, 16, 17, 19, 21, 23, and 24.

Disruptive Behavior during Academics. The following items can be averaged to provide a severity index (ranging from 0 = *not at all* to 3 = *very much*): 4, 6, 13, 15, 20, and 22.

RATING SCALE 3.2. **Parent Academic Management Scale (PAMS)**

Parents: In a typical week, how often did you . . .	0 days	1 day	2 days	3 days	4 days	5 days
1. Use an academic contract or daily rewards program to reward academic habits						
2. Communicate with the child's teachers						
3. Help your child organize school materials						
4. Check to see if your child wrote in a daily planner						
5. Check the grade portal						
6. Help your child plan out what to do during homework time						
7. Help your child do his or her homework						
8. Help your child study for an upcoming test						
9. Check to see if your child had taken notes in class						
10. Monitor whether your child was studying or doing homework when he or she was supposed to be						
11. Use a calendar to help your child plan for an upcoming project						
12. Check your child's homework for errors						
13. Make a checklist or to-do list with your child						
14. Provide a reward for completing schoolwork, homework, or other academic tasks						
15. Restrict privileges for failing to do schoolwork, homework, or other academic tasks						
16. Do some of your child's homework for him or her						
17. In an average week (7 days), I usually spend about _____ hours in activities related to my son's/daughter's academics. (Example responses: 6 hours; ½ hour; 0 hours; 20 hours.)						

(continued)

Scoring and Interpretation

The PAMS can be interpreted by examining individual items to better understand the parent's current level and type of academic involvement. The number of hours the parent spends helping with schoolwork each week also provides an index of the duration of parent academic involvement.

Two indices—EF Oversight (items 3, 4, 6, 7, 8, 9, 10, 12) and Contingency Management (items 1, 11, 13, 14, 15)—can also be calculated by finding the average response value of the set of items on each subscale.

CHAPTER 4

Motivational Interviewing in STAND

The 12th Street After-School Program bills itself as a delinquency prevention program for teens that offers free adult supervision and a range of recreational activities from 3:00 to 6:00 P.M. on weekdays. Inside, adolescents cavort around pool tables, piece together hip-hop dance routines with a local college student, and lie on the ground laughing and talking, sipping vending machine soft drinks. There is a homework room equipped with hand-me-down computer stations, mostly occupied by online gamers and social media checkers. Fourteen-year-old Kelley boards a school bus to the program every day after seventh period, spends 3 hours lollygagging with friends, and meets her mother's minivan in the side parking lot promptly at 6.

Kelley's mother, Diane, arrives at her first STAND session deeply concerned about the traffic. She has driven for an hour to get here. It should have taken 20 minutes. Rush hour is horrible in this city. Kelley drags behind her mother, head down, purposefully tattered sneakers, a tint of blue visible when the fluorescent office lights catch her hair in the hallway. Entering the therapy room, Diane unloads: "I have had it up to here with Kelley. She is disrespectful, untrustworthy, and doesn't seem to care at all about schoolwork. I didn't raise her to be like this. There is something seriously wrong with her brain."

Kelley interrupts her mother. "Excuse me. You are the one who has issues. You are a control freak who wants me to be a cheerleader or something. Everyone I know thinks you are crazy. It's not healthy to be forcing your kid to be perfect all the time. Just let me be myself."

"Is this who you are?" Diane's voice shifts from exasperated to impassioned. "Kelley, you go to the after-school program every day and you are supposed to do your homework there so that when you get home I don't have to deal with you. Yesterday her brother told me that she has been smoking in the woods behind the program. She is very smart but she is in danger of failing eighth grade because she doesn't do any work."

"I do my work! I am not failing any classes right now. I just don't do work when you are around because it's impossible to get anything done with your incessant bird voice. You worry about yourself and I'll worry about myself. This school gives like no homework and I get it all done on the bus. And I'm not smoking, that's just my friends. I just go talk to them because I'm bored."

"This is what I have to deal with," moans Diane.

"Mother, you signed up for this job when you decided to have a child. I am not like you. My grades are fine. If they slip too much I'll pull them up at the end of the school year; it's not hard to do. Coming to see a therapist is a waste of time. It's just another way you try to control me. You spy on me at school by volunteering there every week, you are obsessed with my grades online, and now you think that by taking me here and forcing me to do this program that I will suddenly be like, 'OK, how silly of me, I should start doing all of my work perfectly and become a robot.' "

Diane throws her hands in the air. "This is why you go to the after-school program every day. I can't deal with you. The point of going to the program is for you to get your homework done on your own so we don't have to have these fights. Why don't you just do it? It's not that hard, especially for a smart girl like you." Diane turns to the therapist. "We are here so that you can help Kelley start being more responsible or she is going to fail out of school. She needs to start doing homework."

The Case for MI in STAND

Dyads like Diane and Kelley embody reasons that traditional therapies experience high dropout among teens with attention, EF, or motivation problems. Though both mother and daughter articulate a shared problem (homework problems exacerbated by inappropriate parental supervision), neither enters therapy interested in personal changes—only desiring to see changes made by the other. Kelley feels her mother is overcontrolling and needs to back off. Diane views Kelley as irresponsible and defiant. If Kelley does not agree that she needs to improve her functioning, teaching her compensatory skills would be frivolous. If Diane believes the problem is entirely Kelley's, she is unlikely to make personal changes to her parenting practices. Therefore, desire to make personal changes must be cultivated to ensure a productive therapeutic process.

Motivational interviewing (Miller & Rollnick, 2013) is a counseling style that helps a person decide whether a change is right for him or her. It assumes that making a change is a personal choice that must arise from self-exploration, consideration of one's values and goals, and deciding the best way to act in order to meet these goals and stay consistent with one's values. Like Kelley, many teens in STAND possess goals but may not be fully aware of them. In this case, it is clear that Kelley highly values personal independence and has a strong goal of getting her mother to leave her alone. Diane also appears to value independence (with respect to work completion) and has a goal of seeing Kelley succeed academically. She also has a conflicting goal of avoiding negative interactions with Kelley (more on this later).

Motivational interviewing fits nicely into the philosophy of STAND because it allows these goals and values to be cultivated in a way that catalyzes parent and teen decisions to make personal changes. For teens, it is hoped that STAND's MI components will promote identification of personal goals, increase openness to skill learning and practice, and lay the groundwork for long-term reduction of motivation problems (i.e., helping the teen clearly conceptualize personal reasons to push through boredom and aversive tasks). It also is hoped that MI components will help parents articulate their parenting goals and values, explore the extent to which their current practices support these desires, and empower parents to correct maladaptive parenting habits that inhibit teen growth.

STAND possesses specific therapeutic activities inspired by the MI tradition. The first two engagement modules, as well as the final mobilizing module, are largely MI-focused to plant seeds of change and galvanize maintenance at the end of therapy. Within STAND's skill-based modules, therapists are encouraged to use blended MI that delivers information to families in a style that promotes personal choice and reflection on the benefits of change. Doing so promotes personalization of therapy activities, skill application and practice at home, and family exploration of how new skills will become routine.

The MI Spirit in STAND

The therapist stepping into STAND for the first time may prepare by gaining a basic familiarity with MI. A first step in this process is understanding and connecting with the spirit of MI. As Miller and Rollnick (2013) outline, the MI spirit contains four aspects: partnership, acceptance, compassion, and evocation. Each aspect can be integrated into a STAND therapist's style to enhance quality of treatment.

P·A·C·E·

• *Partnership*. Therapist–family partnership is a critical aspect of STAND. Our assumption is that all parties in the room are equals, each with a unique therapeutic contribution, working toward a common goal. (See Table 4.1 on the next page.)

• *Acceptance*. The MI spirit also includes accepting the parent and teen as they are—often in the face of aversive or irresponsible behaviors displayed by these dyads. In such cases, convincing oneself of the worth of difficult parents and teens can be challenging. The process of acceptance is driven by the practice of empathy—relating to and understanding the experience of parents and teens. (See Table 4.2 on the next page.)

• *Compassion*. With humanistic roots, MI encourages compassion for clients (Miller & Rollnick, 2013)—even when the family's view of success is different from

TABLE 4.1. Partnership

• All parties in therapy room are equals.	• The therapist makes statements to emphasize the autonomy of the parent and teen in therapy.
• Each individual has an important therapeutic contribution.	
• All individuals are working toward a common goal.	• The therapist avoids lecturing, unsolicited advice giving, persuasion, and confrontation.
• Family members are the experts on their own beliefs, goals, experiences, and tendencies.	• The therapist promotes collaborative idea sharing and allows family members to make their own decisions.
• The therapist surrenders the expert role.	

TABLE 4.2. Acceptance

• The therapist sees the unique worth of each parent and teen as a human being.	• The therapist carefully listens to the family's story.
• The therapist affirms worth by focusing on strengths and efforts in therapy.	• Maladaptive behaviors are seen as a natural result of biological and environmental influences.
• The therapist actively practices empathy for the parent and the teen.	• The therapist makes honest attempts to become acquainted with the family.

TABLE 4.3. Compassion

• The therapist accepts that the family's values may be different from his or her own.	• The therapist relinquishes urges to fix the family or depict it as broken.
• The therapist makes earnest efforts to understand the family's best interest, given their personal goals and values.	• The therapist helps the family discover their own path.
• The therapist does not impose his or her own version of success on the family.	• The therapist helps the family practice skills needed to successfully travel their chosen path.

TABLE 4.4. Evocation

• The therapist allows parents and teens to identify their own goals and focus of treatment.	• Family members state their own reasons for trying new skills.
• The therapist asks family members to voice which skills they would like to learn during treatment.	• Family members spend more time in session speaking than the The therapist.
• The therapist encourages parents and teens to personalize the details of home exercises.	• The therapist avoids persuasion.

the therapist's. For example, after extensive values exploration, Diane may decide that she does not wish to increase supervision of Kelley after school because the ensuing conflicts pose a severe threat to Diane's stress level. In this case the parent places the value of a calm home environment above the value of creating structure for the teen. Rather than seeking to convince the parent that monitoring the teen is essential, the therapist may accept that the parent's values are different from the therapist's. (See Table 4.3.)

- *Evocation.* The final aspect of the MI spirit, evocation means drawing reasons and ideas for change from the family rather than imposing a plan for change on parents and teens. (See Table 4.4.)

Resolving Parent and Teen Ambivalence

The parents and teens whom this book is designed to help are a highly ambivalent population. In the case of Kelley and Diane, Diane's ambivalence is striking. One part of her desires for Kelley to succeed in school—chiefly by completing more homework. Another part of her seeks desperately to avoid arguments with Kelley to the detriment of monitoring her homework completion. When she presents for treatment, the desire to avoid negative interactions outweighs Diane's hope for increased homework completion and, ultimately, Kelley's future. As a result, Diane sustains a lack of accountability for homework completion.

MI assumes that most individuals are ambivalent about making changes—to their parenting style, academic habits, or daily routine. With this ambivalence, a part of the family member wants to move forward with the change and another part of him or her holds back, preferring the status quo. The result of this tension can be stasis. No change is made. Without therapeutic components designed to resolve this ambivalence, skill introduction can be fruitless because the parent and teen are not yet ready to try a new pattern of behavior.

Listening carefully to the words of a different kind of ambivalent parent (one who displays a controlling involvement pattern), the therapist hears both sides: "I know I should stop doing his homework for him, it's cheating him of learning opportunities. I'm so scared of what will happen if I do, though. I think his grades will plummet and he will fail the year." *change talk vs. sustain talk*

In this example, the parent's ambivalent statement contains two types of utterances. One is in favor of making the change ("I should stop doing his homework for him") and is coined *change talk*. The other is in favor of keeping the status quo ("I'm so scared of what will happen if I do . . .") and is referred to as *sustain talk*. Change talk and sustain talk represent the two sides of the ambivalence balance.

Change talk takes several forms (Miller & Rollnick, 2013). Preparatory change talk includes utterances that describe a parent's or teen's desire to change, belief in his or her own ability to do so, reasons for making the change, or a sense of urgency surrounding a need to make the change. Mobilizing change talk represents speech that contains the specifics of how change will happen—including commitment language, specific actions planned by the individual, a sense of activation, or steps taken toward the change. Mobilizing change talk typically becomes a focus later in STAND, once the family articulates clear desires for change (see Table 4.5).

The MI process of resolving ambivalence and promoting change is outlined in four overlapping processes: engaging, focusing, evoking, and planning (Miller & Rollnick, 2013). Table 4.6 describes the goals of each MI process in STAND.

The four MI processes intertwine in STAND (see Figure 4.1). For example, in processing the results of a weekly skill experiment, evoking and planning occur simultaneously. The therapist evokes change talk about the benefits of the family's experience and whether it would be worthwhile to continue this skill in the future. With an affirmative answer, the therapist returns to the planning process, asking the family to explore how the skill might be turned into a daily habit that is maintained long term.

Core MI Skills

Miller and Rollnick (2013) detail a set of therapist skills that are employed in MI to support the change process. These skills are relevant whether conversation involves engaging, focusing, evoking, or planning. Core MI skills in STAND are reviewed below and include asking permission, elicit–provide–elicit, open-ended questions, affirmations, reflection, the readiness ruler, and summaries.

TABLE 4.5. Change Talk in STAND

- KELLEY: I'd really like to go to the arts-based magnet high school next year. (Desire)

- KELLEY: I need a C average to be considered for the magnet program. (Reason)

- DIANE: I like this contract idea because once it's written down and signed by both parties, there is less to argue about. I have an idea for something we can try out this week. I think we can make a deal where if she gets her homework done each night, she can go to the after-school program the next day. (Commitment)

- DIANE: Yesterday was a big deal for me. We had an incident where she didn't earn the after-school program and I had to step up and tell her she needed to take the bus home instead of going to the rec center. I didn't argue with her when she protested, just repeated what was stated in the contract. (Taking steps)

- DIANE: I feel like I'm going to have a mental breakdown if she fails this school year. (Need)

- KELLEY: I kept a daily planner for the first couple weeks of this year but then I lost it. I know I could do it again if I felt like it. (Ability)

- KELLEY: I really missed hanging out with my friends at the after-school program that week that I wasn't allowed to. I'm willing to try showing her my homework each night if it means that I can spend time with my friends. (Activation)

TABLE 4.6. MI Process Goals in STAND   E·F·E·P·

Engaging

1. Build therapeutic rapport and working relationship with the family.
2. Understand and affirm family strengths, values, and goals.
3. Communicate a genuine desire to know the family.
4. Ask family members for feedback on initial impressions about the case.
5. Continue a warm, compassionate, and engaging style throughout therapy.
6. Forge a bond with the family to increase their openness to discussing areas of difficulty.

Focusing

1. Narrow targets for treatment with input from the family.
2. Identify clear areas for both parent and adolescent change over the course of therapy. ←
3. Reflect desired changes back to the family to strengthen commitment.
4. Help families prioritize areas for change and formulate a manageable set of treatment goals. ←
5. Encourage separate focusing for the parent and teen to center treatment equally on both. ←
6. Select skill modules from the treatment menu based on mutually selected treatment goals.

Evoking

1. Help parents and teens identify their own reasons for making the change.
2. Elicit change talk from family members and use reflective listening skills to promote elaboration and deepening of change talk language.
3. Minimize instances of sustain talk.
4. Link potential changes to parent and teen goals and priorities.
5. Build self-confidence about making a change through affirmation of efforts and strengths. ←
6. Draw out family member reaction to successes and look forward into the future.

Planning

1. Help family members decide how to put a new skill into action.
2. Elicit ideas for how the environmental structure can be modified to reinforce skill use. ←
3. Use trial runs of each skill to better understand the positive effects of skill use.
4. Detail parent and teen weekly strategy use in parent–teen contracts. ←
5. Process the results of weekly skill experiments to determine how skills can be integrated into a long-term home routine.

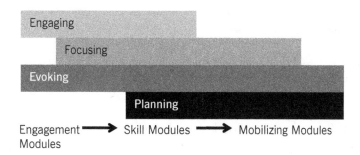

FIGURE 4.1. Parallel MI processes in STAND.

Asking Permission

- The therapist defers control of the session agenda to the parent and teen.
- The therapist arrives to the session with a proposed agenda.

- The therapist promotes family choice during agenda setting by asking permission to conduct proposed exercises and discussions.
- The therapist asks permission to share an idea or suggestion for the family.

THERAPIST: Based on what we talked about last time, I wrote down some ideas for what we could talk about today. Would it be OK if I shared those ideas with you?

DIANE: Sure, go ahead.

THERAPIST: You selected time management strategies as a topic for today. Do those skills still seem like good ones to explore?

KELLEY: Yeah, that's what we chose.

THERAPIST: Great. Well, usually when we do this session with families, we start by discussing what kind of time management strategies you are using right now, and then we can explore some strategies other families have used and talk about which of those strategies might work best for you. How does that sound?

DIANE: That sounds great.

THERAPIST: OK. So then should we start by reviewing last week's skill experiment and then move into the new time management material?

Elicit–Provide–Elicit

- The therapist provides ideas, suggestions, or psychoeducation to the family members in a way that honors partnership.
- The therapist elicits ideas or knowledge from the family before providing a contribution.
- The therapist promotes parent and teen control in the session.
- Parent and teen explore their reaction to the therapist's contribution and are given permission to reject it.

- Across an exchange, <u>the therapist alternates between eliciting information from family members and contributing additional ideas or knowledge</u>.
- The therapist communicates to the teen that he or she is expected to be an active participant in treatment.

THERAPIST: I wonder what you know about effective ways to study for tests and quizzes. (Elicit)

KELLEY: I usually just read it over the night before the test, but I don't know if that's the best way to study.

THERAPIST: You've been trying that method and having some doubts. There are some methods that we've seen other kids your age use that they've told us have been very helpful. (Provide) Would you be interested in having me share some of those with you today? (Elicit)

KELLEY: OK.

THERAPIST: Well, there's a method of studying called active studying. This type of studying involves interacting with the material in a way that forces your brain to process and store it. It usually means doing more than just reading or looking at the material, which some people call passive studying. (Provide) What strategies have you heard of that might fall into the active studying category? (Elicit)

KELLEY: Probably using flash cards and memory tricks.

THERAPIST: Flash cards and memory tricks are exactly right. I'd add to that list taking notes on information that you know you would be tested on. (Provide) What do you think about trying out one or two of those today? (Elicit)

Open-Ended Questions

• Questions that invite families to respond with descriptive rather than one-word answers.	• The therapist should consider the desired type of response before formulating the question.
• Advance the conversation forward and promote change talk.	• Should be used with occasional frequency to avoid an interrogational therapeutic style.

THERAPIST: If things keep on like this, with her not doing any homework after school, how do you see her life looking, say, in one year?

DIANE: I'm really worried that she could fail the school year because of all the missing assignments.

For sample open-ended questions to elicit parent and teen change talk, see Figure 4.2 on the next page.

Affirmations

• Communicate acceptance and empathy to families.	• Powerful for families who are experiencing challenges during the therapeutic process.
• Increase openness to therapist and change.	
• Authentic therapist statements that recognize the strengths, efforts, and successes of the parent and teen.	

THERAPIST: It's been a difficult few weeks for you, Diane, and I know you haven't found a lot of time to do the daily checks you'd hoped to at home. I notice that you've still managed to show up here every week, though, and that really shows a lot of commitment.

DIANE: Thank you, I care about making this work. It's just so hard.

Eliciting Preparatory Change Talk

"What do you hope we can address together?"

"What do you wish for your [teen's] future?"

"What's worked in the past?"

"What kinds of problems are there with the way things are now?"

"How will you know when you are ready to start backing off your homework help?"

"How important is it to you that he or she learn to do things independently?"

"How urgent does this feel to you right now?"

"What would it be like for you if he or she started doing more on his or her own?"

"Suppose these grades continue for the next few years. What do you think will happen?"

"If you had a week off from homework helping, what would you do with that time?"

"What made you decide to choose this module?"

"What kinds of goals do you have for this program?"

"What is important to you as a parent?"

Eliciting Mobilizing Change Talk

"What steps could you take?"

"If you were going to start reducing his or her dependence on it, how would you do it?"

"What ideas do you have for how you can keep an eye on him or her better?"

"How confident are you that you could take one of these steps?"

"Which of these options seem most reasonable for your family?"

"What needs to happen for you to get your grades up to a C average?"

"What do you like about the idea of holding him or her more accountable for his or her actions?"

"What do you think you should do moving forward?"

"How confident are you that you can keep this habit going?"

Planning and Reviewing Weekly Skill Experiments

"What made you decide to select this skill?"

"How do you hope this skill will help you?"

"How can you make this skill fit into your daily routine?"

"What can you do as a parent to promote skill use?"

"How did the daily check-in seem to make a difference?"

"What was the best part about this new skill?"

"How was it for you when you were able to successfully do your homework?"

"You used the skill most days this week—what do you think you'll do moving forward?"

Promoting Long-Term Skill Use

"How is your life different now that you've made these changes?"

"What do you think you'll do if you start to slip back into old patterns?"

"What has it been like for you to see your grades go up?"

"What were your reasons for making this change and sticking with it?"

"What changes do you think you made that supported the adolescent's growth?"

"What do you think you'll do to keep things going as well as they are now?"

FIGURE 4.2. Examples of open-ended questions.

Affirmations should not take the form of cheerleading statements that are nonspecific or overly cheerful or that lack authenticity (see Table 4.7). These may cheapen therapist–family interactions.

Reflections

- Declarative statements that make a guess at what the parent or teen means.
- Statements used to communicate listening and move conversations forward.
- Used strategically to facilitate changes or empathically to communicate understanding.
- Simple reflections represent therapist statements that directly mirror the content of the parent's or teen's speech.

- Complex reflections contain added meaning and often are used to move the conversation toward a particular aspect of the change process.
- There are myriad potential effective reflections for any given statement offered by a parent or teen.

In STAND, reflections are the primary form of therapist–client interaction. The art of forming good reflections develops slowly over time and is summarized at length elsewhere (see Miller & Rollnick, 2013). The therapist is generally encouraged to reflect parent and teen statements in ways that encourage change talk as a response (though there are exceptions to this rule, particularly when communicating empathy during the engaging process). This aim requires therapists to judiciously form reflections that avoid sustain talk responses. Typically, forming reflections that encourage deepened or elaborated change talk require giving preferential reflection to client statements in support of change. Table 4.8 on the next page illustrates the range of reflective statements that can be offered to a single parent or teen utterance.

TABLE 4.7. Affirmation versus Cheerleading

Affirmation	Cheerleading
"Kelley, you found an opportunity to study for your science test on two different days this week. This was the first time trying out this new study skill, and you were able to be successful with it. I'd love to hear about how it went for you on the days you studied."	"Great job, Kelley. You did awesome this week."
"Kelley, you and Mom worked together really well today. You were so respectful to each other during the communication skills activity, it really shows what a strong relationship the two of you are building."	"I think you two are on the ball today!"
"Diane, you've said that increasing accountability is an important goal for you in this program, and by implementing consequences on the days that Kelley didn't do any homework, you really took a major step toward that goal."	"Wow. Way to go this week, Diane!"

TABLE 4.8. Reflecting Parent Change Talk

DIANE: I think its best that I ask her to show me her homework every day before bed, because I don't trust her to tell me the truth if I don't see it with my own eyes.

- THERAPIST: Nightly homework checks could be a way for you to know if she's done it or not. (Simple reflection)

- THERAPIST: Asking Kelley to show you her completed homework each night could help you regain some control. (Complex reflection—guess at unspoken meaning)

- THERAPIST: The proof is in the pudding. (Complex reflection—metaphor)

- THERAPIST: Your worries might let up a little if you had consistent proof that she was doing work. (Complex reflection—describe feelings)

- THERAPIST: Right now you are focused on how you can get involved in a way that supports your daughter to independently complete her assignments. (Complex reflection—reframe)

- THERAPIST: That would be a big triumph for you—to start making nightly checks. (Complex reflection—amplified)

Double-sided reflections are a special kind of reflection that allow the therapist to highlight the change-focused side of a parent or teen's ambivalence.

- The therapist reflects both sides of the parent or teen's ambivalence.
- Two sides of ambivalence are connected with a neutral conjunction (and rather than *but*).
- The second part of double-sided reflection is the side in favor of making change (encouraging a natural response to this component).
- Helpful when family members seem hesitant about trying a new way of doing something or when trying to elicit ambivalence in a headstrong family member.

KELLEY: I'm not sure I need to write down my homework assignments. I think I can remember them on my own.

THERAPIST: Remembering your homework assignments is important to you. Tell me about that.

KELLEY: I don't know. I guess I don't want to have zeros.

THERAPIST: So at this point, one part of you feels like writing down homework is going to be a hassle, and there is this other part of you that really wants to get rid of all these zeros. (Double-sided reflection)

KELLEY: I don't know, I mean I want to get rid of the zeros but I don't know if this is necessary.

THERAPIST: You aren't sure what makes sense for you to do, and you are considering trying to find a way to keep track of work better. (Double-sided reflection)

KELLEY: Yeah, I guess.

The Readiness Ruler

- Sets up an exchange that gauges the parent's or teen's perceived level of readiness for a potential change.
- Asks the respondent to express (on a scale from 0 to 10) how important it feels to make a change.
- Can be employed to query confidence in making a change, likelihood of following through, or willingness to try a new skill.
- Asks the respondent to explain why he or she chose that number—and not a lower one. This follow-up encourages change talk.
- The therapist can provide a second follow-up, asking what is needed to move the respondent to a higher number on the scale.
- Can be particularly useful in STAND when setting up weekly home exercises.

THERAPIST: Diane, on a scale from 0 to 10, with 0 being "not at all" and 10 being "very much," how important is it to you to consistently implement consequences at home when she chooses not to do her homework?

DIANE: Probably a 7.

THERAPIST: A 7. Tell me a little bit about why you picked a 7, and not a 5.

DIANE: I know that I've struggled with consistency and that if I could make some clear rules in the house that it would increase accountability. She really needs a little bit more structure at home. I know it's true.

THERAPIST: A 7 means this is pretty important to you and you have some good reasons to want to hold her more accountable. What would it take to move you up to a higher number on the scale—say a 9?

DIANE: Maybe I'd need to believe that when I set limits with her that it won't turn into World War III. I still really just don't want to get into it with her.

THERAPIST: So you are very interested in being consistent, and most importantly, in a way that will reduce arguments.

Summaries

- A string of reflections that link multiple parent or teen statements.
- Offer clarity to the parent and teen when story is told in new words.
- Can be offered at transition between session topics or at the close of a session.
- Should be concluded with a question that asks family members for feedback on the statement's accuracy (e.g., "Did I get that right?").
- Should be followed with an open-ended question that asks family members to articulate their next step (e.g., "What do you think your next step might be?")

THERAPIST: We spent a lot of time talking about how we could spend the next few weeks together. Diane, you made it clear that helping Kelley pass eighth grade is a priority for you. I got the sense that you really dread the arguments that come up when you ask Kelley about homework. You seem to be looking for a way to hold her accountable for homework without creating conflict at home. You mentioned that reducing these arguments at home, which seem to come up a lot, might greatly reduce your stress level. Did I miss anything important?

DIANE: No, that sounds about right.

THERAPIST: Where would you like to start?

DIANE: I think we need to both agree to some clear rules about homework.

MI in STAND Sessions

Tables 4.9–4.11 on pages 65–66 offer suggestions for MI integration into each phase of STAND.

• The major activities during *engagement modules* are building a partnership with the family, case conceptualization, focusing areas for change, setting treatment goals, choosing skill modules, and introducing parent–teen partnership.

• The major activities in *skill modules* are skill introduction, progress review, planning a weekly skill experiment, and discussing the results of skill experiments.

• The major activities in *mobilizing modules* are to review cumulative lessons learned from weekly skill experiments, planning long-term skill use, and reflecting on positive progress during treatment.

MI Training and Integrity

Without properly delivered MI, STAND reverts to a traditional skills-based treatment that fails to properly engage families and support long-term changes in youth with attention, EF, and motivation problems. As such, for STAND to be delivered with all components intact, the therapist must be properly acquainted with MI. It is recommended that therapists who deliver STAND read Miller and Rollnick's (2013) text and attend at least beginner training in MI to allow for practice of MI skills. A 3-day training is typically recommended to prepare a therapist for basic MI implementation. The Motivational Interviewing Network of Trainers (MINT; *www.motivationalinterviewing.org*) provides ongoing training sessions worldwide with trainers who are vetted for their MI competence and training abilities. We encourage therapists to pursue training offered by a member of MINT. These training sessions are fun and informative and will help MI come to life for attendees.

Following MI training, it is possible to obtain consultation and coaching from MINT members or others who regularly practice MI. Consultation continues the learning process in an experiential way. There are several instruments, the most notable of which is the Motivational Interviewing Treatment Integrity (MITI) instrument, which is in its fourth edition (Moyers, Manuel, & Ernst, 2014). Therapists are encouraged to receive feedback on or self-monitor their MI delivery through such an instrument. Doing so allows the therapist to have confidence that he or she is truly implementing MI.

Self-evaluation can be enhanced by audio-recording sessions and listening to them afterward. When proper permission from families is obtained for doing so, these tapes can be a valuable opportunity for the therapist to evaluate his or her ability using the MI check-ins provided in each session (see Chapters 5–7) or an instrument such as the MITI.

TABLE 4.9. Engagement Modules

Major activity	MI applications
Building a partnership with the family	• Emphasize acceptance, collaboration, and compassion. • Use reflections to communicate empathy and understanding. • Provide affirmations of family strengths and efforts.
Case conceptualization	• Use EPE to provide assessment feedback and information about parenting patterns. • Use summaries to link information gathered in the assessment to new information contributed by the family. • Communicate empathy when discussing difficulties. • Allow family experiences and worldview to drive case presentation. • Emphasize strengths. • Listen for and reflect goals and priorities in favor of positive changes at home and school. • Find opportunities to reflect discrepancies between goals and values and current functioning.
Focusing areas for change, setting treatment goals, and choosing skill modules	• Use change card activity to evoke change talk about reasons for identifying each area for personal change. • Emphasize parent and teen autonomy in setting their own goals for treatment, rather than those desired by another family member (or the therapist). • Use reflections to link treatment goals to desired outcomes. • Use readiness ruler to query the relative importance of each family member's goals. • Listen for and reflect mobilizing change talk about potential steps toward meeting goals. • Use EPE to review treatment menu and emphasize therapist–family partnership when discussing which modules might be most helpful to the family.
Introducing parent–teen partnership	• Elicit change talk about the benefits of creating a parent–teen partnership. • Use EPE to introduce new skills and receive family feedback on how skills might be useful. • Allow family members to personalize their first contract in such a way that emphasizes personal choice in treatment.

TABLE 4.10. Skill Modules

Major activity	MI applications
Skill introduction	• Use EPE whenever new information is to be provided to the family. • Emphasize family choice during sessions to avoid a didactic style. • Elicit change talk about why the family chose a given skill. • Query the family's knowledge about and past experiences with a new skill before introducing it.
Planning a weekly skill experiment	• Allow parents and teens to choose the details of weekly contracts. • Reflect mobilizing change talk about intentions to practice skill. • Ask open-ended questions about contract details to promote parent and teen planning. • Use readiness ruler to query expectations for the home exercise.
Discussing results of weekly skill experiment and progress review.	• Elicit change talks about the benefits of skill use. • Encourage family members to provide their own observations of how the skill was helpful and about lessons learned during the home exercise. • Use an open-ended question to ask the family what they think they will do in the future with respect to continuing the experimental skill. • Use readiness ruler to query the relative importance of each family member's goals. • Communicate empathy when challenges to weekly experiments arise. • Use double-sided reflections to respectfully contrast uncompleted home exercises with previously stated intentions or goals for skill practice.

TABLE 4.11. Mobilizing Modules

Major activity	MI applications
Reviewing lessons learned	• Reframe negative experiences as important learning opportunities. • Ask family members to reflect on what they learned does not work and how they will change the way they do things in response to these lessons. • Integrate these lessons into long-term plans.
Planning long-term skill use	• Query reasons for family choices with respect to using skills long term. Promote elaboration. • Affirm parent and teen successes in integrating skills into new routines. • Listen for and reflect mobilizing change talk.
Reflecting upon progress during treatment	• Affirm positive changes made during treatment. • Offer autonomy support statements attributing progress to specific actions by the parent and the teen. • Build a contrast between the difference between life before and after new parent and teen routines.

CHAPTER 5

Engagement Modules

The purpose of the engagement modules is to prime families for successful skill-based treatment. During these sessions, the therapist makes sincere attempts to understand and develop empathy for the family's circumstances. By unearthing the parent's and the teen's personal goals and priorities, the therapist can collaborate with the family to focus treatment on meaningful and realistic changes.

Parents of teens with attention, EF, and motivation deficits often believe that well-established strategies to compensate for these difficulties are ineffective (see Chapter 1). Their core conviction is that teens will not use compensatory strategies for more than a few days. These observations are valid; with weaker motivation circuitry these teens struggle to initiate and sustain actions that feel tedious and have no immediate payoff. One goal of engagement modules is to increase parent and teen openness to strategies that they may not believe will be effective.

Teens with attention, EF, and motivation deficits display heterogeneous presenting problems. The creeping notion that certain treatment activities are meant for someone else can instill skepticism. Engagement modules emphasize family choice in treatment planning to prevent disengagement.

Like kite flying, therapeutic success in STAND requires both a coordinated initial liftoff and continued guidance to sustain flight. Appropriate collaboration between the parent and teen is critical to both of these processes. Common overcontrolling or unengaged behaviors that emerge after years of parenting an unmotivated or inattentive youth (see Chapter 1) can stymie new attempts to launch treatment skills. Engagement modules provide a safe space for parents to acknowledge their contribution to the teen's difficulties and to increase their openness to making personal changes in support of teen success.

Finally, a successful parent–teen partnership in STAND involves both honest and respectful communication and offsetting teen motivation problems by collaboratively

Engagement Module 1: Understanding the Family. This session reviews assessment results with the family to obtain family feedback on therapist case impressions. By the end of the session, the therapist is able to recapitulate a family-driven case conceptualization that identifies parent and teen strengths and values, areas of teen difficulty, and parenting patterns.

Engagement Module 2: Focusing Treatment Goals. This session considers potential parent and teen areas for change and narrows the focus of treatment to key behaviors that are most meaningful to family members.

Engagement Module 3: Partnership Skills. This session introduces parent–teen skills for collaboration, including staying calm during stressful discussions, listening skills, and expressing oneself honestly.

Engagement Module 4: Creating Structure at Home. This session prepares the home environment for successful skill uptake. This is done by creating a structure in which responsibilities must be completed before the teen can begin enjoyable activities each day.

FIGURE 5.1. Overview of engagement modules.

restructuring the home setting. The parent's primary mission in STAND is to warmly hold the teen accountable for independent skill practice. Engagement modules help the dyad settle into this partnership before skill work begins.

The therapist can move as slowly as needed through the engagement modules—it is OK for a module to take more than one session. Rushing through the engagement process may undermine later success.

Engagement Module 1: Understanding the Family

Checklist for Engagement Module 1

Materials

☐ Notes on earlier assessments (if available)

☐ Visual aids to represent assessment results

☐ Available printouts of adolescent grades or other records

☐ Colored markers, pencils, or crayons

Worksheets

☐ Worksheet 5.1. What's Important to Me Right Now?

☐ Worksheet 5.2. Strengths and Areas of Difficulty

☐ Worksheet 5.3. Parenting Patterns

☐ Worksheet 5.4. Parenting History

☐ Worksheets 5.5 (Parent/Teen). Home Exercise: Into the Future

Topics

☐ Discuss partnership and collaboration.

☐ Complete priorities inventory (Worksheet 5.1).

☐ Build collaborative case conceptualization.

☐ Parent and teen strengths

☐ Teen areas of difficulty

☐ Parenting patterns

☐ Summarize conceptualization and receive family feedback

☐ Introduce home exercise: Into the Future (Worksheets 5.5).

Key MI Skills

☐ Emphasize acceptance, collaboration, and compassion.

☐ Use reflections to communicate empathy and understanding.

☐ Affirm family strengths and efforts.

☐ Use EPE to provide assessment feedback.

☐ Listen for and reflect goals and priorities in favor of positive changes at home and school.

☐ Reflect discrepancies between values and current behaviors.

Case Example for Engagement Module I: Vanessa and Malcolm

Vanessa is a suburban stay-at-home mom who devotes most of her time to shuttling her three kids between school and various activities, housework, and helping with schoolwork. Malcolm is a seventh-grade boy who largely struggles with disorganization and forgetting to complete and turn in homework assignments.

Discussion: Partnership and Collaboration

As described in Chapter 4, one core component of MI spirit is partnership, or the assumption that the therapist and the family members are equals in a shared process of exploring change. This assumption is integral to STAND; as such, treatment can begin with a discussion about the therapist's role in the therapeutic process. Many families will enter therapy with the expectation, based on past experience or common perceptions, that the therapist is an expert who will fix the family's problems. From the outset of STAND, the therapist is encouraged to communicate to family members that change will come from them and that each individual is responsible for choosing to make his or her own changes. The therapist's role is to support this change in whatever ways the parent and teen find helpful.

The therapist should explain that as part of the therapeutic process, both the parent and teen will be asked to consider changes that they would like to make in support of healthy family and school life. It will be up to the parent and teen to decide for themselves whether they will make potential changes. The therapist may emphasize that the more effort the parent and teen put into trying new practices, the more improvement they will experience.

> **KEY POINT: Home Exercise Completion**
>
> The biggest impediment to treatment progress in STAND is failure to practice skills at home as a part of weekly home skill experiments. An upfront discussion with the family about the power of practice communicates to family members that treatment is unlikely to be successful if they decide not to practice techniques at home. The therapist can use MI to explore the family's interest in completing home activities. The goal of this discussion is to increase change talk about actively participating in home aspects of treatment.

During this conversation, the therapist has a first opportunity to try out EPE and MI in the context of STAND. This includes *eliciting* parent's and teen's permission to bring up a topic of conversation, *providing* a small piece of information about STAND, and again *eliciting* the parent's and teen's reaction to the information (see Chapter 4).

Therapeutic Progress

When the therapist introduced the concept of partnership, Vanessa did not expect that she would play a central role in treatment. She also expressed a concern that Malcolm would say what the therapist wants to hear during sessions but would not actually be motivated to participate in therapy activities. The therapist normalized these concerns, mentioning that motivation problems are often a key reason that teens and parents present for treatment. Despite some initial skepticism from Vanessa and minimal participation from Malcolm, the therapist successfully communicated the essence of partnership, laying the groundwork for future therapy activities. The engagement process will continue to unfold for Vanessa and Malcolm over the course of engagement module 1.

5.1 In-Session Exercise: Priorities Inventory

The heart of MI is supporting clients to make personal changes that improve consistency between the client's actions and values. Values and priorities exploration is the first step in this process. Though parents and teens generally know what is important to them, it is not common to reflect upon the relative importance of different aspects of one's life. When the therapist understands parent and teen priorities, he or she is well positioned to support family members as they align their actions with these values. When parents and teens become conscious of their core priorities, they are more likely to act in accordance with their beliefs. These priorities are an important foundation of treatment goal formation. Worksheet 5.1 guides parents and teens to reflect upon their personal values and priorities.[1]

---

[1]All worksheets appear at the ends of chapters.

> **KEY POINT: Encouraging Honesty**
>
> One important aspect of therapy is supporting the parent and teen to be realistic and truthful in session. While identifying core priorities, some family members experience a reflex to select priorities that society may expect of them or that they think the therapist will view as the right answer. In communicating the therapy room as a safe space to share honest viewpoints, the therapist is encouraged to make an explicit statement to the parent and teen about the acceptability of all answers.

During this activity, the therapist presents Worksheet 5.1 as an opportunity for the family members to convey how they are unique. As the therapist understands what is most important to each family member, he or she can affirm and reflect these priorities.

As family members discuss their priorities, the therapist has a first opportunity to evoke preparatory change talk about why the priority area is important to the parent or teen. The therapist can do this by using complex reflections that promote elaboration and deepening of value statements (see Chapter 4). For example:

VANESSA: My two priority areas are helping Malcolm learn how to be more independent and my own mental health. The first one is really important to me because I love him so much and I just want him to grow up to be successful and happy. I'm really worried right now because he needs reminders for everything and I thought this would disappear when he got past elementary school, but some days I think it's even getting worse.

THERAPIST: Your first and foremost priority is your son—especially when he is struggling.

VANESSA: Yes. I make sacrifices. I stay at home to make sure my kids have the best life they can.

THERAPIST: Being present with your kids is a big part of who you are.

As demonstrated below, the therapist can also use open-ended questions (see Chapter 4) to further elicit parent and teen change talk.

THERAPIST: Malcolm, how open are you to sharing what you picked?

MALCOLM: The first one I put was making more friends and the second one I put was not failing the year.

THERAPIST: So two things on the list felt important to you. Tell me about how school is going for you right now.

MALCOLM: Well, I know that at this point it's a possibility that I won't pass seventh grade. I really think I'll pull it off because this happened in sixth grade, too, and I was fine, but it would really be bad if I didn't.

THERAPIST: Passing seventh grade is on your mind a little bit. You suspect you'll be fine, and there is also a part of you that's wondering if maybe you won't be fine.

MALCOLM: I'll probably be fine, but I guess its possible that it could all go wrong.

THERAPIST: Tell me about that possibility—it's got you worried enough to circle passing the year as a priority.

MALCOLM: Well, if you fail two core classes at my school, you get held back. I figured out that I can't pass math—which is fine because I can just do it in summer school. But I also might not pass science. It's not a hard class. I just haven't been doing the work. So I should be fine, but I guess I could still mess up.

THERAPIST: You think turning in more work is going to be critical to passing the year.

Therapeutic Progress

During the values discussion the therapist continued building engagement with the family—particularly with Malcolm, who spoke little during the first part of the session. Malcolm disclosed that his two most important priorities were making more friends and not failing the year. By listening to Malcolm's concerns and giving weight to his priorities, the therapist gave Malcolm a safe opportunity to discuss his difficulties without criticism. The therapist also learned that supporting Malcolm's independence is a very strong priority for Vanessa. The therapist will return to this priority repeatedly throughout STAND, guiding Vanessa to make parenting decisions in support of this value. During the activity, Vanessa also revealed that protecting her own mental health was a current priority for her. She disclosed that she struggles with panic attacks, and the therapist received this information without judgment. Understanding that Vanessa struggles with her own mental health difficulties and wishes to alleviate these symptoms will help the therapist promote changes to her parenting practices in support of this desire.

5.2   Discussion: Parent and Teen Strengths ✪

To promote a strength-based approach to therapy, case conceptualization continues with discussion of teen and parent strengths. Sources of information about parent and teen strengths may include an interview with the parent and teen or teacher reports of the teen's strengths in the school setting (see Chapter 3).

During case conceptualization, information gathered in a preliminary assessment session can be shared with the family, and family feedback is elicited to collaboratively formulate the family's unique story. Depending on the amount of information that was collected about the family prior to engagement module 1, the therapist may spend various amounts of time reviewing already collected information versus eliciting new information.

The therapist can use the EPE approach to offer assessment feedback. The key emphasis in a collaborative, family-driven case conceptualization is not to tell the family how they *are*, but rather to ask the family whether provided information is consistent with their perceptions.

The *strengths* portion of Worksheet 2 allows the parent and teen to take notes on strengths discussed during case conceptualization. The therapist has rampant opportunities to provide affirmations to the family, as well as to evoke continued preparatory change talk about self-efficacy (see Chapter 4). During this conversation, the therapist aims to strengthen the belief that parent and teen strengths will lead them to be successful in treatment.

Therapeutic Progress

During the strengths discussion, Vanessa identified her parenting strengths as being hardworking, always putting Malcolm first, and making sure to spend time with him each week. These strengths were echoed by Malcolm, and, during the conversation, the therapist found opportunities to affirm Vanessa for her parenting efforts— communicating partnership and acceptance. As noted by his math teacher, his mother, and himself, Malcolm's strengths were his kindness to others and sense of humor. As part of this discussion, Malcolm and Vanessa also were encouraged to provide affirmations to each other, promoting a positive parent–teen interaction style in session. *Parent & child affirm one another.*

KEY POINT: Preparing for Assessment Feedback

Collaborative case conceptualization is described in detail in Chapter 3. To prepare for assessment feedback of engagement module 1, the therapist can consult Chapter 3 and arrive to session with written notes on the family, as well as any visual representations of the assessment information that might aid family interpretation of feedback. Doing so helps the therapist prepare for session with an organized set of feedback points to present to the family for EPE-style discussion (see Chapter 4).

Providing visual representations of assessment results in the form of graphs and charts can help facilitate EPE-style discussion and make assessment information seem more objective. Graphs and charts are especially useful when a rating scale or scored test is incorporated in assessment. Offering feedback with visual aids can help parents and teens understand their difficulties compared with others. It is not advisable to bring completed instruments into session, as this may distract from session content and disclose personal information across informants (e.g., some parents may not want their teens to see specific responses to rating scale questions).

Discussion: Teen Areas of Difficulty ✪

Case conceptualization and use of the EPE approach continues with a discussion of the teen's areas of difficulty. Chapter 3 outlines three potential domains of impairment (academics, home behavior, the parent–teen relationship), as well as three categories of deficit (attention, executive functioning, motivation), that are recommended for review during this discussion. For example:

areas to consider

THERAPIST: Would it be OK to discuss some of the areas of difficulty Malcolm is experiencing?

MALCOLM: Sure.

THERAPIST: One area that may be important for us to understand is a domain called executive functioning. I wonder what the two of you have heard about executive functioning?

VANESSA: We've heard about it from his neurologist. I think it has to do with the ability to stay organized and make good decisions.

THERAPIST: Right. Executive functioning is your brain's ability to plan and solve problems and meet your goals. It's kind of like a control panel in your brain. It helps with organizing, planning your time, figuring out what you want to accomplish, and getting yourself to do what it takes to meet your goal. Malcolm, what do you think of that?

MALCOLM: I'm not sure.

THERAPIST: Well, one of the things we know is that people develop their executive functioning skills at different times in their lives. Some people develop them when they are young kids. Other people have to work a little harder and don't develop them until they get to college, or even older. Mom, when do you think you developed some of your executive functioning skills?

VANESSA: I think I started to develop those skills when I was in high school. I remember it was hard for me to stay on top of all of my work in middle school.

KEY POINT: Orienting Families to Key Deficits

When using EPE to discuss attention, EF, or motivation deficits, the therapist may decide to provide basic information on what these brain processes are and how they work; this educational information can help family members understand what is meant by attention, executive functioning, and motivation. As described in Chapter 3, the therapist can begin by asking family members what they've heard about the concept (*elicit*), can provide information about the deficit's meaning (*provide*), and then can ask the family to offer their thoughts on whether the deficit is relevant to the teen (*elicit*).

THERAPIST: That's true for a lot of people. Middle school can be very hard because your school expects you to have some of these skills to succeed, but not everyone has them yet. Malcolm, what do you think about this information I'm sharing?

MALCOLM: It makes sense.

THERAPIST: I have some information to share about what we know about your executive functioning based on the assessment we did last week. Should I share this with you?

MALCOLM: OK.

THERAPIST: Well, keeping track of your homework assignments seems to be one place where executive functioning has been hard for you. Mom and your math teacher mentioned that sometimes you forget what was assigned and sometimes you lose homework before you turn it in. Does that seem right?

MALCOLM: Well, first of all, that teacher is really unfair. But I do have trouble remembering sometimes.

THERAPIST: It's not fun to have unfair teachers, especially when it's a hard class. So one thought might be that strengthening your executive functioning skills, such as organizing and planning, could help you get on top of the homework a bit more. Maybe get that teacher off your back a little. What do you think?

MALCOLM: It seems OK.

The *difficulties* portion of Worksheet 5.2 allows the parent and teen to take notes on areas of difficulty discussed during session. The therapist can allow family members, particularly the teen, to define identified areas of difficulty for themselves. In doing so, the therapist has an opportunity to communicate core aspects of MI spirit—acceptance, empathy, and compassion for the teen. The therapist can find opportunities to evoke preparatory change talk from the teen about his or her desires to make changes to areas of difficulty.

Therapeutic Progress

During the discussion of difficulties, the therapist and dyad openly discussed Malcolm's struggles to keep his school materials organized and to find motivation to complete homework. Initially, Malcolm and Vanessa expressed disagreement about the severity of arguments at home—with Malcolm viewing them as normal to teenage life, and Vanessa seeing them as a significant source of stress. The therapist used graphically depicted objective feedback to highlight the discrepancy between Malcolm's and Vanessa's points of view. Eventually, the therapist found a point of agreement between Malcolm and Vanessa—that homework disagreements start when Vanessa attempts to manage Malcolm's homework; neither enjoys this high level of parental involvement. Using this point of agreement, the therapist suggested that understanding and reducing these disagreements and helping Vanessa reduce her involvement in homework could be potential treatment goals. Throughout the conversation, the therapist listened for mutually noted presenting problems, highlighting them as potential goals for treatment.

Discussion: Parenting Patterns

Continuing with the EPE framework, the final component of case conceptualization is discussion of parenting patterns that influence teen functioning (see Chapter 1) and parenting stress. Sharing data from a parenting stress measure that yields quantitative data about stress level compared with other parents can be especially powerful to parents. Feedback on parental academic involvement may include type and frequency of academic involvement and the total amount of time spent supporting teen academics each week (see Chapter 3). Most support activities are adaptive at certain frequencies and maladaptive at others—a point that should be discussed with the parent. However, the therapist should not label the parent's behaviors as maladaptive.

After reviewing reported involvement behaviors with the parent, the therapist can present Worksheet 5.3. Continuing with EPE, the therapist can share information about the two patterns of parent academic involvement that commonly arise in families when the teen exhibits attention, EF, or motivation problems. These two

---

KEY POINT: Should the Teen Stay in Session?

Depending on the dyad's level of comfort discussing personal issues and the circumstances of the case, it may or may not feel appropriate for the teen to stay in session during the discussion of parenting patterns. The therapist should ask the parent whether or not they would like the adolescent to step out of the room during this conversation. Some parents may feel comfortable discussing their parenting habits and philosophy in the adolescent's presence. Other parents may not. The therapist should be sure to describe the scope of the conversation accurately so that the parent can make an informed decision.

KEY POINT: If the Patterns Do Not Fit

Some parents genuinely do not display the maladaptive patterns described on Worksheet 5.3. Other parents have difficulty recognizing these behaviors in themselves. If the parent does not identify with either of the patterns, the therapist can ask the parent to share a description of any tendencies they've noticed in their parenting that might not be captured by the worksheet—either positive or negative. Worksheet 5.4 can be used to discuss the parent-identified pattern.

patterns (discussed in Chapter 1) are labeled for parents as the *unconnected parent* and the *personal assistant*.

Worksheet 5.4 is a continuation of the parenting pattern discussion. The parent can tell the story of how an identified pattern (maladaptive or not) developed. This discussion includes what factors led the parent to start the pattern, what the parent likes about the pattern, how the pattern causes problems for the teen, and how the pattern causes problems for the parent. This discussion offers an opportunity to evoke preparatory change talk from the parent about desires to make changes to parenting behaviors that may be maladaptive. For example:

THERAPIST: Would it be all right if I shared some information with you about parenting patterns that are common in families when teens struggle with executive functioning problems, like we just talked about for Malcolm?

VANESSA: Yes, of course.

THERAPIST: This handout shows two common patterns that can happen in families. In fact, some research actually suggests that most parents of teens like Malcolm will fall into one of these patterns—at least sometimes.

VANESSA: OK.

THERAPIST: The first one is the personal assistant pattern. It can start happening when the teen isn't getting his work done efficiently or is careless or forgetful. The handout shows that these parents often offer their teens a lot of extra help, check in with the teachers or the grade portal a lot, or provide a lot of reminders.

VANESSA: Well, that sounds familiar.

THERAPIST: You identify with some of that.

VANESSA: Yes. Actually, I can relate to this a lot. I didn't realize it was so common.

THERAPIST: You relate to this idea of helping too much and feeling stuck being a personal assistant to Malcolm. Would it be OK if we explored that pattern a bit?

VANESSA: I've really always had to do this with him, even when he was little. He just was so slow doing homework, and if you left him unattended he would just fiddle with his clothing or watch things going on in the other room. I'd leave him for 20 minutes to do a short worksheet and come back and he would have only written his name on it. So it was always faster and easier for everyone if I just sat down and did it with him.

THERAPIST: This level of help has been going on since the beginning. I suppose Malcolm has really gotten used to it.

VANESSA: He won't even start his homework until I get home now. He says he likes me to help him because he can't focus otherwise. He is right, he can't.

It wasn't a big deal when he was little. But now that he's in middle school, this process is taking hours.

THERAPIST: You'd like to find a way to get him working on his own. That would be a big change to a pattern that's been going on for years.

VANESSA: It doesn't seem like a realistic thing to wish for, but it would be a life changer for us both.

THERAPIST: How so?

VANESSA: I would be able to spend time on my things. With a few extra hours each day?! I could do projects around the house, relax in the evening, and read. Things I haven't done in years.

THERAPIST: You could get some of your personal life back.

VANESSA: Yes.

THERAPIST: So if it's such a strain on your personal well-being, why do you do it?

VANESSA: I guess it reduces my stress, at least knowing he's got his work done for the next day, that we've avoided disaster.

THERAPIST: And what, if any, negative effects have you noticed your level of help has for Malcolm?

VANESSA: Well, for example, I do his online homework for him because it's just easier that way. He isn't getting that learning because I'm doing it.

THERAPIST: And for you? Besides taking your time, how is this high level of involvement problematic for you?

VANESSA: I just am exhausted.

THERAPIST: So let me see if I've got a clear picture of what's been going on for you. Since he was little, you've been providing a lot of homework help and reminders, and now you've got the sense that he's gotten used to this and won't do his work without that level of guidance. You started helping him because—in the moment—it reduced your panic and averted a disaster. Yet, all of this helping is taking a toll on your well-being, exhausting you, and possibly training Malcolm to be dependent on you to get schoolwork done. You worry that it's not realistic to change things at this point—and you would really like to. Does that seem right?

Therapeutic Progress

The therapist used objectively presented information about the frequency and duration of parental academic involvement to elicit Vanessa's reaction to her typical parenting practices. From the objectively presented parenting types, Vanessa identified with the personal assistant pattern. During this conversation, Vanessa disclosed that she often becomes overwhelmed when Malcolm is off-task during homework time and begins to do Malcolm's homework for him. Vanessa offered several pieces of change talk related to her level of exhaustion and concerns about cheating Malcolm of learning experiences when she completes his work. During this conversation, the therapist referred to Vanessa's priority of increasing Malcolm's independence, seeding a discrepancy between her parenting patterns and hopes for Malcolm's development. The therapist emphasized that overinvolvement in academics is common for parents in her position, communicating acceptance to Vanessa. By the end of this discussion, a potential treatment goal for Vanessa is identified—reducing homework helping behaviors.

Discussion: Summarize Conceptualization and Receive Family Feedback

To complete engagement module 1, the therapist should offer an overall summary of the case conceptualization, sharing the major pieces of information emphasized in the session. If the teen left the room for the previous conversation, he or she should be invited to return prior to the case conceptualization summary. As part of the collaborative process, the therapist provides the summary and asks the family for feedback on the summary, revising it as necessary. For example:

THERAPIST: I really enjoyed our meeting today. I learned a lot about the two of you. Malcolm, you are a smart young man who is seen as very respectful to others and whom everyone says is really witty. Right now you are having some trouble in math and science that is threatening your ability to pass seventh grade, and that's been on your mind a little bit. You are thinking you'll pull it off, but you're not sure, and so you might be open to some new ways of approaching work in those classes. You'd also like to find ways to connect with other kids your age locally because those friendships are something you really feel like you are missing out on. Does this sound right so far?

MALCOLM: Yeah.

THERAPIST: Mom, you care tremendously about your son's future and will give anything to help him succeed—including much of your free time and a lot of your emotional investment. You try hard to build in fun activities on the weekend so that you can keep a positive relationship with your son, and, at the same time, the hours of homework help, doing work for Malcolm, and arguments that come out of the pushing and prodding are starting to add up. You mentioned lately you've been worrying now about your own mental health. You also said you were desperate to find a new way to support Malcolm—one that emphasizes his independence because you are a little worried that he's missing out on some opportunities for learning and growth when you are the one managing homework. You aren't convinced there is another way, but you are interested in finding out what's possible. Did I get most of that right?

VANESSA: That sounds about right.

Parent Content: Using the subgroup discussion format, parents can be prompted to discuss their impressions of (1) teen strengths, (2) parent strengths, (3) teen areas of difficulty, and (4) parenting patterns. As part of the parenting patterns discussion, the therapist can distribute Worksheets 5.3 and 5.4 and ask parents to consider the information contained on these worksheets.

Teen Content: Teens can also be prompted to discuss their strengths and areas of difficulty. Using a large-group format, the therapist can list these areas on a board to facilitate sharing and to communicate that teens in the group may share common difficulties and strengths. As part of this discussion, the therapist can introduce the concepts of executive functioning and motivation. The therapist can ask teens to discuss how difficulties in these areas may lead to problems at school and at home.

Collaborative Content ✪: As part of a collaborative exercise, parents and teens can be encouraged to share their impressions of parent and teen strengths and areas of difficulty. This conversation can occur in private dyads throughout the group room. At the end of the private dyadic discussion, parents and teens may volunteer to summarize their conversations to the full group.

FIGURE 5.2. Delivering engagement module 1 in a group.

Home Exercise: Into the Future

The therapist can direct the parent's and teen's attention to Worksheets 5.5. During the next week, the parent and teen each can be asked to write a description about how she or he would like her or his life to be in 3 years, following the prompts on the worksheet. The purpose of this activity is to help parents and teens visualize their hopes for the future, strengthening the importance of achieving these dreams.

Engagement Module 2: Focusing Treatment Goals

Checklist for Engagement Module 2

Materials

- ☐ Completed change cards (see Chapter 3)
- ☐ Extra blank note cards
- ☐ Colored markers, pencils, or crayons

Worksheets

- ☐ Worksheet 5.6. Personal Goals
- ☐ Worksheet 5.7. Menu
- ☐ STAND Worksheets 5.8 (Parent/Teen). Home Exercise: Letter from the Future

Topics

- ☐ Discuss hopes for three years in the future.
- ☐ Complete change cards activity.
- ☐ Set goals for treatment.
- ☐ Select skill modules from menu.
- ☐ Introduce Home Exercise: Letter from the Future (Worksheets 5.8).

Key MI Skills

☐ Evoke change talk related to personal changes.

☐ Emphasize parent and teen autonomy in setting their own treatment goals.

☐ Use reflections to link treatment goals to desired outcomes.

☐ Use readiness ruler to query relative importance of goals.

☐ Reflect mobilizing change talk about potential steps to meeting goals.

☐ Use EPE to review treatment menu and select skill modules.

Case Example for Engagement Module 2: Hope and Jenna

Jenna is a 16-year-old student at a large public school who is repeating ninth grade after ceasing all academic work at the end of the previous school year. Hope is Jenna's aunt, who adopted her at the age of 3. Hope maintains little interest in providing academic support or guidance for Jenna at home, believing that she is too old for homework help.

Discussion: Three Years in the Future

The therapist can begin the session by reviewing the home activity. The family members are asked to share their hopes for 3 years in the future. As they do, the therapist can listen for preparatory change talk regarding desires to change the status quo (see Chapter 3). When preparatory change talk is detected, the therapist can use reflections and open-ended questions to deepen change talk and promote elaboration. In particular, the therapist can build a discrepancy between how life is currently and how the parent and teen hope life will be in the future. As a demonstration, we join Hope and Jenna at the tail end of this discussion.

THERAPIST: So, Jenna, you've mentioned that in the next 3 years you'd like to see yourself getting good grades so you can go to college, develop good relationships with your teachers, and find ways to get involved in activities with other kids.

JENNA: Yeah.

THERAPIST: That's different than how things are now. How so?

JENNA: Well, right now, even though it's the beginning of the school year, my grades are already bad. I have mostly C's and D's. Also, I'm not very popular, and my teachers basically hate me.

THERAPIST: You'd like to find a way to bring your grades up, become closer with your teachers, and form more friendships.

JENNA: Yeah.

THERAPIST: What do you think it would take to make that a reality?

JENNA: Um, I think I would need to do better on tests at school and focus more.

As far as friends go, I really want to be friends with more people at school, but I don't really know how to do that.

Therapeutic Progress

Jenna began the discussion by reading her worksheet out loud—disclosing that in 3 years she hopes to make straight A's, have teachers who appreciate her, be considered popular in school, and have a boyfriend. The therapist probed why strong grades and positive relationships with teachers were important to Jenna, learning that she hopes to go to college. The therapist also learned that Jenna has an interest in being permitted to participate in more social activities—a piece of information that may be key to helping Jenna find motivation to complete schoolwork as treatment continues. The conversation also allowed the therapist to elicit change talk from Jenna about needing to do better on tests and focus more during class to improve her grades. During this discussion, Hope reveals a strong desire to see Jenna graduate from high school so that she can avoid some of the negative life events that Jenna's biological mother experienced. This piece of change talk is also critical—discussing this desire may be a key to building Hope's motivation to become a more involved parent when it comes to academics.

In-Session Exercise: Change Cards ✪

Using the information gathered in the assessment session and discussed in engagement module 1, the therapist should arrive to engagement module 2 with a completed set of change cards. The process of creating these cards between engagement modules 1 and 2 is described in detail in Chapter 3.

The change card activity is designed to help families review potential areas for change and narrow their focus for treatment into distinct meaningful areas (see Figure 5.3). Note cards are used to represent each potential area for change in order to create a visual representation of these domains that can be physically manipulated for ranking their importance. As discussed in Chapter 3, change cards represent potential areas of change for both the parent and the teen, and the number of change areas identified for each should be relatively equal.

KEY POINT: Parent-Focused Changes

Some parents may be surprised that change cards also involve parent-specific areas for change. They express the belief that all change during STAND should come from the teen. The therapist should be careful not to perpetuate this belief during the change card activity. Parent and teen changes should be emphasized to an equal extent. As changes are prioritized, the therapist should ensure that the conversation balances discussion of parent and teen areas for change, rather than solely focusing on teen deficits.

Step 1: Introduce the change card exercise by asking permission to review some potential areas for change that were mentioned by the family in engagement module 1.

Step 2: One card at a time, offer each potential area for change to the family members, making separate lists for the parent and the teen.

Step 3: Emphasize that only the family members will be able to decide what kinds of changes might be right for them and encourage the family to remove cards from the list if not relevant.

Step 4: Ask family members to add any cards to the list that seem to be missing. Listen for and reflect preparatory change talk about the importance of each potential area for change.

Step 5: Ask family members to consider the relative importance of each change on their personal lists. Encourage the family to use colored markers to highlight whether a change is *priority, high priority,* or *urgent.* Each family member should determine the colors for his or her own list. Link reasons for change to hopes for the future articulated by the family earlier in the session.

Step 6: Listen for preparatory change talk indicating a need or sense of urgency for a change. Take the time to ask for elaboration on urgent areas, promoting discussion of where this sense of urgency comes from.

FIGURE 5.3. Steps for conducting the change card activity.

When the change card activity closes, there will be a range of potential change areas that can be targeted during STAND. Each family member agrees that these changes are priorities and has a clear sense of *why* these changes are important when the therapist links these changes to each family member's hopes for the future. Next, the process of linking potential changes to desired outcomes continues by setting shorter-term goals—objective achievements to be met by the end of treatment.

Therapeutic Progress

After completing engagement module 1, the therapist created five change cards—three for Jenna and two for Hope. These cards were:

1. Find ways to prepare for tests. (Jenna)
2. Get homework done in a shorter period of time. (Jenna)
3. Remember what was discussed in class. (Jenna)
4. Find ways to promote Jenna's independence. (Hope)
5. Create structure at home that encourages homework completion. (Hope)

The case conceptualization revealed that for years Jenna has done poorly on tests—partly because she rarely studies for them, partly because she doesn't retain information presented in class, and partly because she has trouble understanding concepts. Another consequence of her poor retention and comprehension is that it takes her a very long time to finish homework. Thus, identified areas for change (for Jenna) target study skills, note taking in class lectures, and reducing time spent on homework.

Hope rarely monitors or reinforces Jenna's schoolwork, believing that 16-year-olds should be self-sufficient. Thus Hope's areas for change include finding ways to promote Jenna's independence and increasing structure at home (which will require an increase in her involvement). Using words such as *independence* and *structure* when discussing change cards increases Hope's buy-in because they match her belief that Jenna should be required to complete responsibilities without assistance.

During the change card activity, Jenna agrees that test preparation and increasing homework efficiency are important treatment goals; however, she disagrees with the card about remembering what was discussed in class. The therapist asks Jenna whether she would be willing to keep the card on the list, and she obliges. To respect Jenna's insistence that the card did not fit, the therapist focuses conversation on the cards with which Jenna agrees.

Although Hope continues to state that Jenna should independently manage her own academic work, she concedes that improving structure at home could help Jenna focus. The therapist will continue to reflect Hope's desire for Jenna's independence when she later introduces the idea that responsibilities should be completed before relaxing and fun activities are enjoyed (engagement module 4). To close this discussion, the therapist asks Jenna and Hope to reflect upon how these potential changes might help them meet their long-term goals.

In-Session Exercise: Treatment Goals

Following the change cards activity, the therapist can direct the family's attention to Worksheet 5.6, which provides space for the parent and teen to articulate goals for themselves over the duration of treatment. In helping family members set these goals, the therapist can emphasize that:

- Goals should be meaningful—something each family member would personally like to see change in his or her own habits.
- Goals should be realistic next steps that can be accomplished by the end of treatment.
- Parents and teens should each set separate goals for their respective selves—most importantly, parent goals should surround parenting behaviors rather than teen behavior.

Once goals are formulated, the therapist can use open-ended questions and reflections to evoke change talk surrounding reasons for desired changes (see Chapter 4). By deepening change talk, the therapist helps family members strengthen their commitment to changes being considered. As part of this process, the readiness ruler

> **KEY POINT: Collaborative Family-Focused Process**
>
> The concern returns that some parents will attempt to make treatment teen-focused, rather than family-focused. Some parents will set goals for themselves that are actually goals for the teen (e.g., see her or him study more frequently, have her or his grades improve). In these cases, the therapist should offer gentle corrective feedback that the goals are supposed to be personal. Similarly, it is important for the therapist to create a space in which the teen can form his or her own goals, rather than being influenced by the parent. Sometimes teens have trouble thinking of or articulating a goal. Parents who are accustomed to prompting or helping the teen may offer suggestions to the teen, who may accept these suggestions in an effort to complete the activity faster. The therapist can protect against this possibility by reminding the teen of past change talk he or she has offered, clarifying instructions for the teen, or simply by being patient while the teen takes time to articulate goals.

(see Chapter 4) can be useful to query the parent or teen's perceived importance of and confidence in meeting goals. For example:

THERAPIST: Hope, your first goal is to find ways to promote Jenna's independence. What made you choose that goal?

HOPE: I see that she gets off the hook about not doing her homework when I get busy with all of my responsibilities and don't always check to see if she has done hers.

THERAPIST: You'd like to build into your day a way to check in on her—and do it every day.

HOPE: Yes.

THERAPIST: And on a scale from 0 to 10, with 0 being not at all and 10 being very much, how important is it to you to improve how you hold her accountable?

HOPE: Oh, it's high, probably a 9.

THERAPIST: A 9. Why did you pick that number, and not say, a 5 or a 6?

HOPE: Well, I think that she needs to get into shape and its time we had more rules around the house about what is acceptable and what is not.

THERAPIST: You'd like a clear plan for how she's going to get her work and studying done, and what's going to happen if she does and doesn't.

Therapeutic Progress

During the goal-setting exercise Jenna states that her three goals are to get B's or higher on tests, make more friends, and get homework done more quickly. In asking her to elaborate on her choices, the therapist learned that Jenna felt demoralized after recently learning that she has the lowest average in her class, which made her want to pull her grades up to avoid embarrassment. The therapist used scaling questions to query Jenna's readiness to make changes in these areas, learning that she very much wants to do better in school but is only somewhat confident in her own ability to do so. This information helped the therapist to understand that increasing Jenna's self-efficacy through affirmative therapeutic interactions, providing Jenna with the necessary skills to succeed, and increasing accountability for Jenna's practice of these skills will each be an important component of treatment.

Reluctantly, Hope indicated that she thinks she could be more consistent and wants develop a more positive relationship with Jenna. Her third goal was somewhat dogmatic—she restated that she is not interested in checking up on Jenna. The therapist verbally reframed this goal as setting clear expectations for independence, but Hope remained steadfast in her goal's wording. Shifting focus, the therapist continued to link these goals to Hope's disclosure that she worries that Jenna will travel on a similar path as her biological mother.

In-Session Exercise: Skill Module Menu

With areas for change identified and initial goals set, the treatment-focusing process is under way. This process continues with selection of individualized skill modules. In partnership with the therapist, the family selects modules from a list of seven options, linking skill modules to their goals for treatment (Worksheet 5.7). The therapist can present the menu to the family and review each choice with the parent and the teen, making sure they understand the content of each module.

Using EPE, the therapist can elicit from the family any modules that seem fitting, can provide (with permission) advice on which modules best match the family's stated goals, and can elicit a final decision from the family on which modules might be best.

KEY POINT: *Choosing Skill Modules*

It is suggested that skill modules be limited to three in number—at least at first. Mastering a few new skills typically serves the teen better than introducing six or seven new skills, leaving limited opportunities to focus on mastery of each. The teen becomes spread too thin with this high level of skill introduction.

The Writing Down Homework and Making a Homework Plan modules build two foundations for homework success: knowing what the homework is and clarifying how the home environment should be structured to promote homework completion. As such, mastery of the skills presented in these modules is typically necessary to improve homework problems. The therapist should suggest these modules, first and foremost, if the teen has difficulty keeping track of homework assignments or if the family seems to lack a consistent or distraction-free homework routine. Many of the other modules are difficult to conduct without the homework skills being in place. This is especially true for Time Management Strategies and Study Skills.

KEY POINT: *When the Family Selects Modules That Seem Like a Poor Fit*

If a family selects a module that seems counterintuitive given their previously articulated areas of change or goals, the therapist may choose to query the discrepancy and ask for elaboration. The therapist can also ask permission to share concerns about module choice, given work with prior families. Ultimately, however, the autonomy of the family should be honored in selecting their own skill modules after the advice of the therapist is given and the family's rationale is discussed. It is always possible to revisit choices with the family later when the focusing process further unfolds.

We rejoin Hope and Jenna for their discussion of skill modules.

THERAPIST: I wanted to look ahead with you both to the next few weeks of this program and talk about different skills you might want to focus on. Would that be OK?

JENNA: Yeah.

THERAPIST: Because every family is different, you have some choices to make about what we spend our time doing.

HOPE: OK.

THERAPIST: This handout is called a menu, and it contains seven different skills we might spend time on during this program. Would you like me to go through what each of the seven choices is all about?

HOPE: I think we can read it.

Hope and Jenna stare at the menu and ask occasional questions about the modules. Once each component has been clarified, the therapist continues:

THERAPIST: So when you look at the list, which of these skills jump out at you?

JENNA: I think we should do the study skills one since that is the main goal on my list.

THERAPIST: That seems like an obvious choice to you.

HOPE: What about the time management one because that might help you get through your homework more easily?

JENNA: I think note taking would be better.

THERAPIST: A few jump out at you. Would it be OK if I shared with you some of my thoughts based on what we've talked about so far? You are certainly free to reject them, since you know yourself best.

HOPE: Of course.

THERAPIST: So when there are homework problems, the first thing we usually check is whether the teen knows what the homework is each night. This usually involves keeping a daily planner or having a really organized school homework website that you can check. How is Jenna doing in this area?

HOPE: She has a homework website that she goes to. So that isn't an issue for us.

THERAPIST: Great, so then the second thing to check is whether everyone is on the same page about a clear plan for homework time. How do you feel about this area?

HOPE: That is definitely still a problem area for us.

THERAPIST: OK, so you may want to consider the module on making a homework plan.

JENNA: OK, then, what about if we do that one and also the study skills and the note taking?

THERAPIST: Those three modules definitely seem to support your goals. Hope, how are you feeling about those choices?

HOPE: I'm not really sure. I guess it's OK for now, though.

Therapeutic Progress

In reviewing the treatment menu, Jenna expressed an immediate interest in the study skills and note-taking modules. Hope believed that the time management module might be most useful to Jenna, but Jenna seemed to disagree. With permission, the therapist suggested that the family complete the homework plan module because this skill would support their goals of increasing consistency at home and getting homework done more efficiently. Jenna and Hope momentarily agreed with the therapist's logic, and these three modules were selected. At the close of the session, the therapist made a mental note to revisit Hope's continued skepticism in subsequent sessions.

All group sessions begin with a joint home activity review from last session.

Parent Content: Using the subgroup discussion format, parents can be prompted to: (1) create change cards for themselves, (2) prioritize change cards using the color-coded system, and (3) set end-of-treatment goals for themselves. As part of this discussion, the therapist can distribute Worksheet 5.6.

Teen Content: Teens can also be prompted to create and prioritize change cards for themselves and discuss end-of-treatment goals.

Collaborative Content ✪: Parents and teens can collaborate to create a finalized list of change cards that reflects both parent and teen areas for change. The parent and teen can each provide feedback on the others' card lists and prioritization, adding or removing cards as needed. Parents and teens can also discuss their goals for treatment.

FIGURE 5.4. Delivering engagement module 2 in a group.

This effort may include reflecting change talk that links potential parenting changes to her one strongly stated goal—to prevent Jenna from following in the footsteps of her biological mother.

Home Exercise: Letter from the Future

The therapist should direct the parent's and teen's attention to Worksheets 5.8. The parent and teen should be asked to each write a letter to his or her present self from his or her future self in 3 years. In this letter, the parent and teen should offer advice to their present selves for meeting the goals that were set in engagement module 2. The purpose of this activity is to help parents and teens mobilize toward taking actions in support of making potential changes to their habits.

Engagement Module 3: Partnership Skills

Checklist for Engagement Module 3

Materials
- ☐ None

Worksheets
- ☐ Worksheet 5.9. Staying Calm
- ☐ Worksheet 5.10. Communication Skills
- ☐ Worksheet 5.11. Planning a Parent–Teen Meeting

Topics
- ☐ Share advice from future self (Worksheets 5.8)
- ☐ Discuss parent–teen partnership
- ☐ Staying calm during stressful situations at home
- ☐ Reflective listening
- ☐ "I" statements
- ☐ Home Exercise: Planning a Parent–Teen Meeting (Worksheet 5.11)

Key MI Skills
- ☐ Evoke change talk about the benefits of parent–teen partnership.
- ☐ Use EPE to introduce partnership skills.
- ☐ Link the benefits of partnership skills to stated treatment goals.

Case Example for Engagement Module 3: Leah and Robert

Robert is a ninth-grade male who lives with his mother, Leah, and his older sister. Leah works a strenuous job in finance and complains that she cannot oversee her son's academics because her career requires her to be accessible to the office at all times. Robert expresses that his mother frequently criticizes him for not completing his work and bringing home bad test grades but states that his grades are equivalent to those of his peers. Leah also explains that Robert lies about his homework completion, tries to hide his grades from her, and is often disrespectful to his teachers. Robert denies these claims.

Discussion: Share Advice from Future Self

The therapist can begin the session by asking family members to share their letters from the future. During this conversation, the therapist can listen for mobilizing change talk embedded in the letters (see Chapter 4). This mobilizing change talk may include statements about actions or steps that promote goal achievement. When reflecting change talk, the therapist should reinforce the link between potential changes, engagement module 2 goals, and engagement module 1 priorities. The purpose of this discussion is to strengthen commitment to goals and identify ways to meet them. When reviewing letters from the future, the therapist should emphasize *personal* changes that the letter writer might make in support of goals (rather than allowing parents to focus on changes the teen should make—or vice versa).

After Leah reads her letter from the future, her therapist discusses it with her.

LEAH: I said in the letter that I would support him to improve his grades, but to be honest, I'm not so sure there's anything I can do at this point. He needs to wake up and realize that he is ruining his own future.

THERAPIST: You mentioned in the letter you might want to be tougher with him. I'd like to hear more about that.

LEAH: I know it sounds like the right thing to do, but I'm just worried that it won't work.

THERAPIST: You think it sounds like the right thing to do—to set some limits together.

LEAH: He's lazy and I've taken everything away and nothing seems to matter to him.

THERAPIST: You aren't confident that you can come up with a reasonable structure together, and at the same time, I get the sense you are open to trying anyway.

LEAH: Yes, I suppose that's true.

THERAPIST: Why?

LEAH: Well, we are here because things are getting worse every day. If you think something will help, then I'll definitely try it.

THERAPIST: And if something you tried worked, how would that improve your quality of life?

LEAH: Then I would be less angry with him.

THERAPIST: You'd feel a lot less stressed.

LEAH: If he started doing his part, I would definitely be less stressed.

THERAPIST: So let me see if I'm on the same page. You think that setting some limits together could be a way to improve the structure at home for Robert. You worry a little that keeping a daily structure isn't possible in your case. And yet, you are willing to give it a try in case it helps him get more done—because that would have a big impact on your stress level. Did I get it right?

Therapeutic Progress

Robert and his mother each shared their letters from the future. In her letter, Leah imagined Robert opening an acceptance letter from a prestigious college. She described how Robert's hard work earned him teacher respect and recognition. Leah described a more relaxed household and indicated that she might need to change the structure at home to encourage Robert to start doing more homework. In summarizing Leah's letter, the therapist emphasized the link between creating structure at home and reduction of Leah's stress—something that is a stated priority for her. Robert's letter was fairly simple and focused on improving his homework problems so that he would make better grades in school. As a result, the therapist attempted to elicit greater detail from Robert—particularly about reasons he might want to improve his school grades.

Discussion: Parent–Teen Partnership

Using EPE, the therapist can engage the parent and teen in a discussion about the meaning of partnership and what skills they believe are necessary to form a successful partnership. The therapist can explain that parent–teen interactions can be strained when there are homework difficulties or when the parent has difficulty finding ways to motivate or support the teen. The family members can be encouraged to discuss their relationship, including its strengths and how they would like to see it improve. The therapist can emphasize that many activities in STAND will require them to work together at home and can ask the family's permission to spend the session discussing how to strengthen their partnership.

In-Session Exercise: Staying Calm during Stressful Situations at Home

The therapist can explain that stressful situations often arise when the teen struggles in school. Both the parent and teen can experience strong emotional reactions to these situations. Referring to Worksheet 5.9, the therapist can ask the parent and teen to each list two situations related to academics or the parent–teen relationship that lead them to feel upset or angry with each other. During this process, the therapist can normalize the family members' examples, explaining that their examples are common for families. Figure 5.5 is an example provided by Robert and Leah.

After discussing the situations, the therapist can ask the family members to consider the benefits of staying calm during these situations. During this exercise, the therapist can listen for and reflect change talk about controlling emotions to enhance communication and problem solving, staying respectful to one another, and other benefits identified by family members.

Completion of Worksheet 5.9 can continue by asking family members to each list two things they can think and two things they can do to help themselves stay calm in these situations. Figures 5.6 and 5.7 present two examples.

Parent: Describe Two Stressful Situations	Teen: Describe Two Stressful Situations
1. When I come home and Robert hasn't even started his homework.	1. When my mom doesn't believe me and I'm telling the truth.
2. When I find out Robert has lied to me about something.	2. When my mom starts yelling at me for something normal (like getting a C on a difficult test).

FIGURE 5.5. Sample responses to Worksheet 5.9.

Parent: What I Can Think to Stay Calm	Teen: What I Can Think to Stay Calm
1. It's not worth getting upset over this.	1. Just stay calm. She doesn't know the whole story.
2. If you react when he lies, he's just going to lie even more.	2. Don't let her get to you and ruin your day.

FIGURE 5.6. Sample responses to Worksheet 5.9.

Parent: What I Can Do to Stay Calm	Teen: What I Can Do to Stay Calm
1. Take a deep breath and count to 3.	1. Think about a song I like in my head and listen to that instead of the yelling.
2. Go into another room until you are calm and then go talk to him about it.	2. Write down what I'm mad about instead of saying it to my mom.

FIGURE 5.7. Sample responses to Worksheet 5.9.

> **KEY POINT: Reflective Listening**
>
> Reflective listening means listening to what the other person says and taking a guess at what he or she means. Just as reflections are used in MI to help the client feel heard and understood by the therapist, family members can use reflective listening to improve their communication during discussions. Just as in therapy, good reflections take the essence of what the other person said and offer a rephrasing back to the speaker rather than parroting the speaker's exact words.

In-Session Exercise: Reflective Listening ✪

The therapist should introduce this exercise by explaining that partnership takes clear communication between the two people involved to make sure both people understand each other. Using EPE, the therapist can elicit ideas from the family about particular communication skills that could be used to build a successful partnership. If no ideas are given by the family, the therapist may explain that the ability to make sure you understand the other person (reflective listening) is the first skill. See Figure 5.8 for examples.

Good Examples

PARENT: My goal is to be able to give you fewer reminders because I want you to do things more independently.

TEEN: You are going to try to stop giving me so many reminders because you think that will help me learn to do things on my own.

- -

TEEN: My goal is to do my homework every night so that I don't have so many missing assignments.

PARENT: You'd like to have fewer missing assignments so you are going to try to do better with your homework.

- -

Poor Example with Therapist Corrective Feedback

TEEN: My goal is to get A's on all of my tests and quizzes by the end of the year because I want to be a good student.

PARENT: Do you really think that's possible? I don't think that is a very realistic goal for you to have. Why don't you change it to a C average on your tests? That might be more realistic.

THERAPIST: Mom, is it OK if I offer you some feedback on your reflection?

PARENT: Sure.

THERAPIST: I could tell that when you heard what he said, you remembered something we talked about before, which is keeping goals realistic. So that was a smart thought. How did you think you did with providing a reflection of what he just said?

PARENT: Yeah, I guess that wasn't really a reflection. That was just my opinion.

THERAPIST: Would you want to try again and give a reflection this time? Do you feel prepared to do that?

PARENT: Sure.

FIGURE 5.8. Examples of reflective listening.

The therapist can ask family members to consider how reflective listening might be useful to them. When introducing this skill, the therapist can refer to Worksheet 5.10. The therapist can model reflective listening for family members by asking one of them to share a goal that they have for therapy and why they chose that goal. The therapist can reflect back the family member's point in a demonstration. For example:

ROBERT: My goal is to turn in more homework so that my mom stops bothering me so much.

THERAPIST: You've decided to focus on completing your homework because you think doing so will get your mom off your back.

Once the family appears to understand the meaning of reflective listening, they can begin their own practice of this skill. The therapist can ask permission to offer an activity that would allow for reflective listening practice.

The parent and teen can practice reflective listening using the therapy goal topic demonstrated by the therapist above. The parent and teen can alternate sharing goals for therapy while the other practices reflective listening. With permission, the therapist should offer feedback to the parent and teen on their reflective listening skills and continue practice until both demonstrate the skill correctly.

In-Session Exercise: "I" Statements ✪

The therapist can introduce "I" statements as the second partnership skill. Using the same EPE format, the therapist should ask the family members what they've heard about "I" statements and share the meaning of "I" statements as needed. Worksheet 5.10 may serve as a guide. See Figure 5.9 for examples.

The therapist can demonstrate an "I" statement by telling a brief story (true or fictional) about a situation that occurred in which the therapist disagreed with someone. The therapist can first offer what he or she might have said (inappropriately) and can then offer what he or she said instead ("I" statement). This juxtaposition allows family members to see the difference between how people typically

---

KEY POINT: "I" Statements

"I" statements are a way of respectfully communicating disagreement with another person. "I" statements are a way to focus your opinion on how you feel, rather than what you disagree with. "I" statements follow the following format:

I feel _____ when _____

because _____.

react to disagreement and how an "I" statement improves communication. For example:

THERAPIST: The other day I got upset with my neighbor because he keeps parking in my front yard and I finally saw him and wanted to say something about it.

ROBERT: What did you say?

THERAPIST: What I wanted to say to him in my head was: "Get out of my yard. Why would you think that's appropriate!? You are selfish to think you can just park in someone else's yard!"

ROBERT: That would be funny.

THERAPIST: But I'm not looking to start a fight with my neighbor. So I used an "I" statement instead. I said: "I feel kind of bothered when you park in my yard because that's my only space to park and I need it for my own parking."

Good Examples

Parent "I" statement: I feel exhausted when I have to keep nagging you about homework because it doesn't ever seem to do any good.

Teen reflection: You get tired of always bugging me about homework.

- -

Teen "I" statement: I feel annoyed when you always yell at me to start my homework because usually I'm already doing it and you didn't even check.

Parent reflection: You don't like me yelling at you about homework because you feel like I'm not noticing when you've already started.

- -

Poor Example with Therapist Corrective Feedback

PARENT: I feel angry when your teacher calls me in to talk to me about your homework because that's your problem and you are being lazy and I've told you a million times to do it and you just don't listen. She needs to be talking to you, not me.

THERAPIST: Mom, is it OK if I offer you some feedback on your "I" statement?

PARENT: Sure.

THERAPIST: You started out great with naming the emotion you were feeling and describing when it happened. It seemed like when you got to the part about why you felt that way, you started to get angry again.

PARENT: You bet.

THERAPIST: One of the goals of "I" statements is to express your opinion in a way that focuses on what you feel, rather than what you disagree with about the other person. How did you think you did with that part of it?

PARENT: Yeah, I guess maybe I got a little carried away.

THERAPIST: Do you want to try again?

PARENT: Sure.

FIGURE 5.9. Examples of "I" statements.

ROBERT: That's nicer.

THERAPIST: How do you think the neighbor would react differently to the two statements?

ROBERT: I think he would get angry in the first one. In the second one, he might be more likely to be polite and move his car.

Following the therapist's example, the family can be prompted to think of an issue about which they disagree and to each use an "I" statement to communicate their perspectives. With permission, the therapist can offer corrective feedback to the parent and teen until the skill is demonstrated correctly. The therapist can also prompt the family members to use reflections to mirror each others' "I" statements.

Therapeutic Progress

Robert and Leah initially struggled with the skills of reflective listening and "I" statements, requiring consistent corrective feedback from the therapist. When they began to get angry during the session, the therapist referred back to Worksheet 5.9 and the techniques they each identified to stay calm during discussions. The therapist also openly asked the family to consider why the communication skills felt difficult to them. Both agreed that they felt easily angered by the other, and the therapist reflected and normalized this concern, eliciting change talk from the family members about practicing the techniques discussed in session in order to strengthen their relationship.

Home Exercise: Parent–Teen Meeting

The therapist should direct the family to Worksheet 5.11. The therapist can explain that the home exercise for the next week is holding a parent–teen meeting to discuss progress on their goals. The therapist should elicit the family's reaction to the

---

All group sessions begin with a joint home activity review from last session.

Parent Content: Using the subgroup discussion format, parents can be prompted to (1) discuss situations with the teen that lead them to become angry, (2) identify coping skills for dealing with this anger, and (3) introduce the concepts of reflective listening and "I" statements.

Teen Content: Teens can also be prompted to discuss situations that lead them to become upset with their parents, coping skills for dealing with this anger, and the skills of reflective listening and "I" statements.

Collaborative Content ✪: Parents and teens can meet in dyads to practice the communication skills (reflective listening and "I" statements). Following the communication skills activity, parents and teens can plan a meeting for the upcoming week.

FIGURE 5.10. Delivering engagement module 3 in a group.

exercise and ask the family members to imagine how the meeting will go and to discuss which skills they will practice in support of a successful meeting. In planning the home exercise with the family, the therapist can ask the family to discuss the benefits of holding such a meeting, reflecting their responses to strengthen offered change talk. Family members should be encouraged to practice staying calm, reflective listening, and "I" statements during the meeting.

Engagement Module 4: Creating Structure at Home

Checklist for Engagement Module 4

Materials
- ☐ None

Worksheets
- ☐ Worksheet 5.12. Current Structure at Home
- ☐ Worksheet 5.13. Parent–Teen Contract

Topics
- ☐ Share experience with parent–teen meeting
- ☐ Explore current structure at home
- ☐ Introduce idea of choosing responsibilities first
- ☐ Create a parent–teen contract
- ☐ Home Exercise: Implementing contract

Key MI Skills
- ☐ Evoke positive experiences during past week.
- ☐ Use EPE to introduce concept of putting responsibilities first.
- ☐ Strengthen openness to this strategy by reflecting its perceived benefits.

Case Example for Engagement Module 4: Sam and Michael

Michael is a sixth-grade male who lives with his parents and younger sister. He participates in STAND with his father, Sam, who describes himself as the parent who supervises homework. Michael's mother works evenings, and Sam returns home by 5:30 P.M., at which point he prompts Michael and his sister to begin homework while he prepares dinner. Sam explains that after dinner, he asks Michael to join him in the living room to finish his homework. Sam states that Michael needs constant supervision during homework time or he will play games on his computer instead of doing his work. Sam adds that his homework involvement includes helping Michael answer questions, checking his work for him, and watching to make sure he does not play computer games. During engagement module 2, Michael's articulated goals for treatment were to write down his homework assignments in a planner, keep his book bag clean, and have no missing assignments at school. Sam's goals were to provide less assistance to Michael on homework assignments, to find ways to motivate Michael to complete work independently, and to hold him accountable for not playing games during homework time.

Discussion: Share Experience with Parent–Teen Meeting

The therapist can begin the session by asking the parent and teen to describe their experiences with the parent–teen meeting. During this discussion, the therapist should reflect positive experiences while holding the meeting, including all attempts to practice engagement module 3 skills. Review of the home exercise can close by querying what the parent and teen hope to do in the future to continue communication skill practice. For example:

THERAPIST: You both decided to hold a parent–teen meeting this week to discuss your goals. How did it go?

SAM: It didn't go that well, to be honest. We started yelling at each other within 2 minutes.

THERAPIST: You found time to hold the meeting—that's great, some of the families we work with forget.

SAM: We held it like we planned, on Saturday afternoon. It just ended up making us more stressed out, though, to talk about the goals because he is still struggling with everything.

THERAPIST: It can be really hard to hold a calm discussion about stressful topics. Which of the skills we talked about last week did you two try out?

SAM: Well, I think we both tried to use the listening skills and the "I" statements at first. But once we got angry, we stopped.

THERAPIST: You remembered the communication skills we talked about and even got a few tries in.

SAM: Yeah, it seemed like the conversation was going well at first, to be honest. Then I think we just both got upset.

THERAPIST: One thing you learned is that once someone gets angry, you both become upset and it becomes harder to use those skills.

SAM: Yeah, I think we need to take a time-out next time if things start to go that direction—because it's not productive.

THERAPIST: You remembered to hold the meeting, got a good 2 minutes of skill practice in, and had a really important insight this week—which is that if you can both stay calm, you actually communicate pretty well. Where do you think this leaves you?

SAM: I think we need to keep practicing ways to stay calm when we are talking with each other.

THERAPIST: You'd like to get to a point where things are naturally calmer, and you see practice as the key.

Therapeutic Progress

As demonstrated above, Sam initially maintained that the home exercise was a failure due to an argument that broke out during the parent–teen discussion. The therapist carefully reflected the positive elements of the exercise, and Sam began to articulate what was useful about their experience during the last week. By the end of the exchange, Sam agreed that continuing to practice communication skills could be a key to improving his relationship with Michael. After eliciting Sam's experience with the home exercise, the therapist learned from Michael that he enjoyed the beginning of the meeting with his father but felt blamed for his homework problems as the meeting progressed. Michael stated that he would be open to another meeting and suggested they suspend the meeting if anyone got emotional with the other person.

In-Session Exercise: Current Structure at Home

The therapist can introduce the activity by stating that creating healthy structure at home includes designating appropriate times to complete responsibilities and enjoy relaxing activities. To explore the family's current structure at home, the parent and

Fun or Relaxing Activities	Responsibilities
Teen	Teen
Eat snacks	Homework
Play video games	Feeding the dog
Watch TV	Cleaning my room
Texting	Reading
Going online	Studying
Shopping	Taking out the trash
Playing soccer	Brushing my teeth
Parent	Parent
Watching TV	Bills
Having a beer after work	Cleaning
Checking social media	Supervising teen's homework
Calling relatives on the phone	Church leadership
Playing poker	Cooking

FIGURE 5.11. Brainstorming activities and responsibilities.

teen can complete Worksheet 5.12, an inventory of the responsibilities and relaxing or fun activities that the parent and teen currently spend time on at home. Part of Worksheet 5.12 lists sample responsibilities and fun/relaxing activities for the teen to help him or her build a list. See also Figure 5.11 on page 99 for examples.

Following completion of Worksheet 5.12, the therapist can prompt the family to discuss how long they currently spend on activities on each list and the extent to which they adequately balance enjoyable activities with responsibilities. Engaging the parent in this exercise is a way to help the parent understand the benefit of putting responsibilities before fun or relaxing activities.

Discussion: Creating Structure That Puts Responsibilities First

Using EPE, the therapist can explain that structure at home can sometimes be rearranged in a way that helps the teen master his or her responsibilities. As part of this discussion, the therapist can offer the idea that requiring responsibilities to be completed prior to relaxing activities can promote independence by making expectations clearer to the teen. As part of this dialogue, the therapist can introduce the idea that knowing that relaxing activities must wait until after responsibilities can create motivation to complete responsibilities that seem hard or boring. The therapist can ask the parent and teen to share their thoughts on creating this kind of structure at home.

Continuing with EPE, the therapist can close the discussion by probing the teen's openness to trying the responsibilities-first structure during the upcoming week. The therapist can suggest that the teen choose one responsibility and commit to putting it before all fun or relaxing activities on the list. The therapist can explain

---

KEY POINT: It's Not Bribery or Privilege Removal—It's Structuring

Some parents express a concern that putting responsibilities before fun or relaxing activities feels like bribing the teen for something he or she should be doing naturally. Other parents complain that removing privileges does not motivate the teen. In differentiating bribery and privilege removal from creating a structure that puts responsibilities first, the therapist may decide to discuss the following:

- By putting responsibilities first, the parent and teen are deciding to rearrange the day's structure so that enjoyable activities in which the teen already partakes must wait until after responsibilities. This is a natural rearrangement that can motivate the teen.
- Choosing to introduce new rewards into the teen's environment is not a part of this activity. Removing privileges as a reaction to teen failure is not, either.
- The teen should be engaged in determining which enjoyable activities he or she is willing to suspend until responsibilities are completed.
- Teens with attention or motivation problems often develop internal motivation (the ability to self-motivate) much more slowly than his or he peers do. Creating a structure that requires responsibilities to occur before relaxation time is a way to help teens compensate for motivation difficulties while internal motivation continues to develop.

that the purpose of this experiment is for the teen and the parent to evaluate whether putting responsibilities first improves structure and balance at home for the teen. During this discussion, the therapist can emphasize that the experiment lasts only 1 week and that the family is free to continue or discontinue the structure afterward.

Therapeutic Progress

During the discussion of putting responsibilities first, Sam explains that he uses this technique on himself every evening by waiting to watch TV until after he has finished cleaning the kitchen. Michael agrees that the concept of putting responsibilities first is logical and says that he would be willing to try it for 1 week. After affirming the family's openness to the strategy, the therapist reiterates that the fun activities must be the things that Michael already does on a regular basis—not new privileges.

In-Session Exercise: Using a Contract to Make a Plan

Using Worksheet 5.13 as a guide, the therapist can show the parent and teen a sample parent–teen contract that makes a plan for this week's home exercise. Using EPE, the therapist can elicit their reaction to the contract as a tool for making a plan.

As part of this exercise, the therapist can guide the parent and teen to complete a contract that includes (A) the teen's daily responsibilities in the plan, (B) a list of activities that must wait until after the daily responsibility is completed, (C) what the parent will do to reinforce the contract, and (D) how the parent will ensure the teen completes responsibilities independently (without parental assistance).

Discussion of the parent's role in the contract (parts C and D) is critical. For the contract to be successful, the parent should be prepared to monitor the teen's

---

KEY POINT: Removing Reminders and Help to Promote Independence

It is logical for parents to believe that the best way to help teens follow a contract is to remind or help them. However, when parents provide a lot of help and reminders, teens may learn that they do not need to complete responsibilities independently because a parent will prompt and help them to do so.

In addition, parents become exhausted by constant reminding and helping and may start to believe that the teen is incapable of completing the task independently. Afraid to stop prompts and helping for fear of the teen's failure, they keep reminding and coaxing.

In place of reminders and helping, the parent can politely inform the teen that he or she has not yet earned relaxing activities if the teen attempts to access them prematurely. Parent–teen contracting often involves a retraining process. The teen learns that he or she must complete responsibility without help or reminders. The parent must learn to resist the urge to interfere and to muster the strength to withhold from the teen what he or she wants but has not yet earned.

access to fun activities once he or she arrives home from school—and to step in if the teen attempts to access privileges prematurely. This may include holding on to the teen's phone after school, storing away video game controllers, or restricting websites through parental controls. The therapist should conduct a thorough discussion of these steps with the parent, probing his or her readiness to monitor the teen's activities after school. If the parent offers logistical barriers to doing so, the therapist should engage the parent in brainstorming about ways to overcome these challenges.

Here, the therapist discusses Sam's involvement in the contract.

THERAPIST: Sam, what do you view as your role in this contract?

SAM: I can remind him to feed the dog when we get home.

THERAPIST: You think a reminder would be a good way to get involved, and yet, I remember that you said you had a goal of wanting Michael to be a little more independent than he is now with his responsibilities.

SAM: That is true, but without a reminder, I'm not sure we are going to get very far.

THERAPIST: I'd be happy to share an idea that families in the past have used, if you'd like?

SAM: Of course.

THERAPIST: Instead of reminding, families who are concerned about dependence sometimes make an effort to supervise the teen's access to relaxing activities as soon as he or she gets home. If the teen tries to engage in one of the fun activities, the parent simply says "you haven't earned that yet." How would that approach fit with your parenting?

SAM: I think that could work. So I just have to make sure he can't get on his electronics after school. I guess I'm going to have to hold onto a few things until he feeds the dog.

THERAPIST: How doable does that seem to you?

SAM: I think I can do it.

THERAPIST: And if Michael decides not to feed the dog one evening?

SAM: I guess I'll just keep holding on to them.

Once the contract is complete, the parent and teen can sign it.

Therapeutic Progress

In negotiating the contract, Michael suggests that his responsibility be feeding the dog. Michael explains that he chose feeding the dog as his chore because it is something his father always nags him to complete. Sam initially says that his role in the contract will be to remind Michael to feed the dog. The therapist points out that a

All group sessions begin with a joint home activity review from last session.

Parent Content: Using the subgroup discussion format, parents can be prompted to (1) discuss balance at home, (2) make an inventory of responsibilities and relaxing activities they complete at home, and (3) discuss how putting responsibilities before fun activities may improve motivation.

Teen Content: Teens can also be prompted to discuss the concept of finding balance at home and make an inventory of their daily responsibilities and relaxing activities.

Collaborative Content ○: Parents and teens can create a parent–teen contract as displayed in Worksheet 5.13.

FIGURE 5.12. Delivering engagement module 4 in a group.

reminder may prevent Michael from practicing the skill of being self-directed. As a result, Sam agrees that he will not provide reminders to his son. They decide that Michael will not access his list of fun activities until he feeds the dog and that Sam will support Michael by monitoring his electronics use and only allowing him access to these activities when he shows proof that the dog is fed.

Home Exercise: Implementing Parent–Teen Contract

The therapist should ask the parent and teen how they feel about implementing their parent–teen contract during the next week. In doing so, the parent and teen should discuss how implementing the contract might improve balance at home for both of them. Beneath the contract in Worksheet 5.13 is a log for documenting whether the parent and teen each did their part in the contract.

Parent (pick two)

My job	My mental health	Teen's social life	Respect
My health	Teen's success in sports	Other family members	Personal freedom
Our finances	Spirituality or religion	Preparing teen for college	My marriage or relationship
Teen's passing year	Promoting teen's independence	Leisure activities	Avoiding conflict with teen
Teen's getting high grades	My social life	Community service	Other:

Teen (pick two)

Doing my best in school	Finding friends	Video games	Shopping
Being popular	Success in sports	Pleasing my parents	Personal freedom
Making money	Spirituality or religion	Being ready for college	Boyfriend or girlfriend
Passing the year	Doing things without help	Having more fun	Avoiding conflict with parents
Getting high grades	Getting to do more things with friends	Community service	Other:

Teen Strengths:

Parent Strengths:

Teen Areas of Difficulty:

When a teen struggles with attention, executive functioning, or motivation problems, a parent often responds in one of two ways.

Parent Avoids or Gives Up

Parent Overly Assists or Controls

Teen lacks accountability at home for work completion.

Teen can become dependent on parent help or reminders to complete work.

The Unconnected Parent
• Becomes disengaged from teen's academics.
• Expects adolescent to work independently.
• May believe it is pointless to work with the teen.
• Sometimes is too busy or tired to pay attention to teen.
• Often unaware of adolescent's grades until report card.

The Personal Assistant
• Can become overly involved in teen's schoolwork.
• May sit with adolescent during homework time.
• Communicates heavily with teachers.
• Frequently checks grades online.
• May often ground adolescent or remove privileges.
• Sometimes does homework for the teen.
• Worries that teen will fail without high support.

Pattern I relate to:

Why this pattern got started:

Why the pattern has not stopped yet:

Problems this pattern causes for the teen:

Problems this pattern causes for me:

In 3 years, what do you really hope your life will be like?

What would a typical day be like for you?

What parenting accomplishments from the past 3 years would you be most proud of?

What would your family and social relationships be like?

What would your relationship with the teen be like?

What else do you hope for 3 years in the future?

In 3 years, what do you really hope your life will be like?

Will you still be in school? If so, where?

What will your life at school be like?

What will your interactions with others your age be like?

What will your relationship with your parents be like?

What will you do for fun?

Look ahead to the end of our time working together. What goals would you like to see yourself accomplish?

Consider goals that are realistic to achieve and would be meaningful to you.

Parent Goals for Self	Teen Goals for Self
1.	1.
2.	2.
3.	3.

Skill Modules
_____ **Writing Down Homework** Work together to make an action plan for keeping track of what the teen's homework assignments are each night. This module will help with forgetfulness about homework and can empower parents to know what the teen is supposed to be working on.
_____ **Making a Homework Plan** Work together to set mutual expectations for where, when, and how homework should be completed each night. Set clear limits on the parent's involvement in homework and what activities have to wait until after homework is completed.
_____ **Organization Checkups** Work together to set expectations about how school materials should be stored and organized. Plan regular organization checks and what to do if the teen passes the checks.
_____ **Time Management Strategies** Learn a strategy to help you get started on work when you dread it because it is hard or boring. Learn how to schedule homework tasks using a method that increases time on task during homework.
_____ **Study Skills** Learn study skills techniques that are particularly helpful for teens with attention or executive functioning difficulties. Work together to make a study plan for an upcoming test that breaks up studying over several days.
_____ **Note Taking** Decide on how you might use note taking to improve your attention in class and relationship with your teachers. Work together to make a plan in which the parent provides accountability for taking notes at school.
_____ **Problem Solving** Learn decision-making skills that help you slow down and think through challenging situations, choosing a solution carefully. These skills can be helpful when troubleshooting why a skill listed above is not working for you.

In the space below, write a letter from your future self in 3 years to your present self. Your future self should tell you what it is like to meet your goals as a parent.

1. Describe how you are parenting in the future and how you feel about it.
2. Explain what steps you took to become this type of parent.
3. Give your present self some advice.

Dear Present Parent,

_____

_____

_____

_____

_____

_____

_____

_____

_____

_____

_____

_____

_____

_____

Sincerely,
Future Parent in 3 Years

In the space below, write a letter from your future self in 3 years to your present self. Your future self should tell you what it is like to have met your goals and what advice you have about what to do to get there.

1. Describe what you are doing in the future and how you feel about it.
2. Explain what steps you took to get to your future.
3. Give your present self some advice.

Dear Present Self,

_____

_____

_____

_____

_____

_____

_____

_____

_____

_____

_____

_____

_____

_____

_____

Sincerely,
Future Self in 3 Years

_____

Parent: Describe Two Stressful Situations	Teen: Describe Two Stressful Situations
1.	1.
2.	2.

Parent: What I Can Think to Stay Calm	Teen: What I Can Think to Stay Calm
1.	1.
2.	2.

Parent: What I Can Do to Stay Calm	Teen: What I Can Do to Stay Calm
1.	1.
2.	2.

Reflective Listening: Guessing at someone's point

Example:

PARENT: My goal is to be able to give you fewer reminders because I want you to do things more independently.

TEEN: You are going to try to stop giving me so many reminders because you think that will help me learn to do things on my own.

I Statements: Communicating disagreement respectfully and honestly

I feel _____ when _____

_____ because _____

_____.

Example:

TEEN: I feel annoyed when you always yell at me to start my homework because usually I'm already doing it and you didn't even check.

PARENT: You don't like me yelling at you about homework because you feel like I'm not noticing when you've already started.

Plan a meeting during the next week. The topic of the meeting will be to share with each other your progress on goals that you set.

When will the meeting be held? _____

How will you remember to hold the meeting? _____

What skills will the parent use to stay calm and clearly communicate during the meeting?

What skills will the teen use to stay calm and clearly communicate during the meeting?

Typical Fun or Relaxing Activities	Daily Responsibilities
Teen	Teen
Parent	Parent

Sample Fun or Relaxing Activities

		Sample Daily Responsibilities
Texting	Staying up late	Feeding pet
Video games	Watching Netflix	Doing dishes
Listening to music	Computer games	Taking out trash
Using phone	Social media	Completing homework
Driving	Riding bike	Writing down homework
Drying or straightening hair	Working out	Cleaning room
Walking home with friends	Playing instrument	Studying for test
Going online	Watching TV	Completing online learning
Sports	Taking a nap	Working on a project
Shopping	Chatting with friends	Making bed
After-school activities	Playing games or cards	Taking a shower
Spending time with boyfriend or girlfriend	Hanging out with friends	Being ready to leave for school on time

Sample:

(A) **Teen daily responsibility:** *Feeding the dog*

(B) **Teen list of enjoyable activities that must wait until after responsibility is completed:** *Computer games, TV, phone, tablet*

(C) **Role of parent in reinforcing part (B):** *Hold onto teen's phone when he gets home until he feeds dog. Make sure he doesn't use other electronics until he feeds dog.*

(D) **To promote independence, what the parent will *not* do:** *Won't provide any reminders. Won't give a lecture if he forgets.*

(A) **Teen daily responsibility:**

(B) **Teen list of enjoyable activities that must wait until after responsibility is completed:**

(C) **Parent role in reinforcing part (B):**

(D) **To promote independence, what parent will *not* do:**

_____   _____
Teen Signature   Parent Signature

	Did teen do (A)?					Did parent do (C & D)?				
Day:	1	2	3	4	5	1	2	3	4	5
Y/N?										

CHAPTER 6

Skill Modules

The purpose of skill modules is to introduce compensatory strategies that help the teen overcome cognitive deficits in attention, EF, or motivation. Brain research suggests that these deficits likely persist throughout an individual's lifetime (Shaw et al., 2006), and available treatments do not yet permanently correct neurobiology. The good news is that individuals can permanently improve the way they function at home, school, work, and with others, even though deficits remain.

The class of cognitive deficits treated in STAND is multifaceted. Each teen typically displays a subset of these difficulties, which means some skill modules will be helpful to the teen and others will not. To cover the range of deficits displayed by these teens, skill modules address problems with memory, motivation, planning, staying focused, organizing oneself, and being thorough. After identifying the most helpful strategies, the teen can work to forge habits that promote lifelong compensation for cognitive deficits.

For teens, mere introduction of skills is typically insufficient to promote long-term strategy use. Consistent practice is needed so that strategies become second nature to the teen. Age-appropriate adult oversight is imperative to ensure that the teen practices independently. During skill modules, parents also practice new strategies to master their own role in this process: (1) eliminating prompts, reminders, and helping behaviors that prevent independent skill practice, (2) structuring the home environment so that enjoyable activities must wait until after teens complete responsibilities, and (3) staying consistent and firm while placing limits on freedoms when teens do not complete responsibilities as promised.

After skills are introduced, parents and teens mutually devise a practice plan for the upcoming week: Teens make plans for independent skill use, and parents make plans for age-appropriate oversight. This plan is outlined in contract form (see engagement module 4 in Chapter 5) each session.

Seven skill modules are outlined in this chapter. Based on the teen's areas of need, families are encouraged to select sessions from the treatment menu introduced in engagement module 2. Each skill module follows the same four-part format: (1) review skill use during the past week, (2) introduce a new skill, (3) discuss how the skill can be introduced into the family's home routine, and (4) create a plan for practicing the new skill during the next week.

Structure of the Universal Skill Module

All modular sessions follow the same structure, as detailed below. Following this section, the unique content of each skill module (1–7) is presented in succession.

Checklist for the Universal Skill Module

Universal Topics

☐ Review of last week's skill experiment

☐ Progress review

Skill Module 1: Writing Down Homework: Discuss current attempts to remember homework. Strengthen commitment to remember homework. Make a plan for recording homework (with parent monitoring and contract).

Skill Module 2: Making a Homework Plan: Discuss current homework habits and goals for homework completion. Strengthen commitment to improve homework completion. Create plan for homework time with parent monitoring component. Implement parent–teen homework contract.

Skill Module 3: Organization Checkups Discuss current organization habits and goals. Strengthen commitment to improve organization. Establish organization system for (e.g., book bag, bedroom) and document on checklist in Worksheet 6.7. Establish parent–teen contract for monitoring organization.

Skill Module 4: Time Management Strategies Introduce concept of prioritization. Discuss use of checklists for task completion and breaking tasks into small components to overcome motivation problems. Discuss parent's role in monitoring task completion and planning out tasks (e.g., homework time). Create sample to-do list.

Skill Module 5: Study Skills Discuss current test performance and study habits. Introduce active versus passive studying. Flash cards and notes from text activities. Create study plan with parent monitoring component. Strengthen commitment to change test scores.

Skill Module 6: Note Taking Discuss current practices for retaining material presented in class. Identify benefits of note taking. Provide instruction and feedback on sample notes. Create a contract for note taking during upcoming week with parent monitoring component.

Skill Module 7: Problem Solving Discuss goal for problem solving and factors that contribute to the problem. Brainstorm solutions and discuss pros and cons of each solution. Outline implementation of selected solution (using contract as needed). Strengthen commitment to plan.

FIGURE 6.1. Overview of skill modules.

Step 1: Elicit change talk from teen about perceived benefits of using the new skill. Pay particular attention to affirming the adolescent's successes during the past week, even if they were small.

Step 2: Listen for change talk from teen about reasons to continue skill use. Reflect these statements appropriately to strengthen teen's commitment to skill practice.

Step 3: Elicit change talk from parent related to reinforcement of the practice plan and allowing the teen to perform skills independently. Redirect conversation as needed to affirm the parent's successes during the past week, even if they were small.

Step 4: Listen for change talk from parent about reasons to continue their efforts. Reflect these statements to appropriately strengthen parent's commitment to skill practice.

Step 5: Ask the parent and teen to consider whether they will continue skill use past the 1-week period. As part of this conversation, the therapist can ask about reasons for continuing skill use, as well as about the details of how long-term skill use might occur—including how the parent hopes to continue monitoring and reinforcement of skill practice.

FIGURE 6.2. Steps for conducting a successful home exercise review.

☐ Introduce skill

☐ Create practice plan

☐ Introduce this week's skill experiment

Key MI Skills

☐ Use EPE to present information to family.

☐ Emphasize family choice in designing practice plans.

☐ Elicit change talk about any positive choices or behaviors during past week.

☐ Reflect mobilizing change talk about intentions to continue parent and teen skills.

☐ Use readiness ruler to query perceived importance of new skills and confidence in implementing them.

☐ Communicate empathy when challenges to weekly skill experiments arise.

☐ Use double-sided reflections to respectfully contrast uncompleted home exercises with previously stated intentions for skill practice.

Discussion: Review Last Week's Skill Experiment

The core elements of skill experiment review involve assessing the extent to which (1) the teen practiced the new skill during the past week, (2) the parent reinforced teen practice by maintaining a responsibilities-first structure at home, and (3) the parent allowed the teen to practice skills independently by refraining from reminders and helping. See Figure 6.2 for steps for conducting a review. Throughout these discussions, the therapist should use key MI skills to strengthen family members' commitment to continued use of successful strategies (see Chapter 4).

KEY POINT: Incomplete Home Exercises

When home exercises are not completed, the onus typically falls upon the parent for not initiating his or her end of the contract. Some parents do not follow through on their portion of the weekly skill experiment. Unless the therapist probes, some parents are not forthright about their nonparticipation. Therapists are encouraged to ask specific questions to parents about whether they monitored teen skill use each day, whether they were able to hold back reminders and help, how they responded to adolescent skill utilization, and how they responded when the adolescent failed to use the skill. To promote an open therapy environment, the therapist should communicate empathy when the parent discloses that he or she did not do his or her part. Conversation should focus on affirming any small efforts made by the parent and the parent's intention to follow through with plans in the future.

When parents or teens report problems executing a weekly skill experiment, the therapist should refrain from promoting sustain talk about what went wrong—particularly when the parent blames, confronts, or complains about the teen. Instead, the therapist should frame skill experiment review to discuss what the parent and teen learned from the experience and how they will modify skill use to overcome barriers to skill practice.

During the home experiment review, it is important for the therapist to help families grasp the relationship between teen skill use and parental efforts (e.g., reinforcing a structure that puts responsibilities before enjoyable activities, withholding reminders). The therapist may ask the parent to specifically comment upon how she or he believes her or his actions influenced the teen's skill use during the past week.

If the family decides not to continue skill use, the therapist can develop a discrepancy between goals that relate to the practiced skill and the decision to cease skill practice. The therapist can ask parents and teens to clarify this discrepancy and offer ideas about what will help them meet the goal in the absence of skill practice. However, ultimately it is up to the family members to determine whether a skill feels helpful to them. Following is an example of a typical home exercise review in STAND, in which the parent and teen follow their skill contract partially. For this example, we return to our high-conflict engagement module 3 dyad, Robert and Leah.

THERAPIST: Last week, the two of you made a plan for Robert to practice writing in a daily agenda and for mom to check Robert's agenda each day after school and only allow access to electronics in the evening after he had shown mom the agenda. Should we start by hearing how it went?

LEAH: I've had it up to here with him. He only wrote in the planner on 2 days. And it's the same thing as always. These plans just don't work for him. He is too lazy.

THERAPIST: OK, I hear that you are disappointed that the plan didn't go as smoothly as you hoped, and yet it sounds like there were a couple of good days in there. Maybe we can hear more about those days.

LEAH: Well, 2 days out of 5 isn't exactly successful.

THERAPIST: Robert, why don't you walk me through your decision to write down homework on those 2 days?

ROBERT: Well, I'm happy to write in the planner if she would follow her part of the plan, but she didn't check anything until the car ride right before we got here today, so what's the point, exactly?

LEAH: Excuse me. You are old enough to be handling this on your own. You know I have to work, and you need to learn to step up.

THERAPIST: So if I've got this right, Robert, you started to write in it for 2 days and you are interested in continuing the skill but are hoping mom will find time to do the checks you two planned out.

ROBERT: She won't do it.

THERAPIST: And so when you thought she was going to check it, you wrote down your homework last week, but when you realized she didn't have time to, you stopped.

ROBERT: She needs to do her part.

THERAPIST: Leah, it sounds like you were able to get a check in before coming into the session, so that's a step ahead of a lot of families.

LEAH: It was the week from hell for me. I admit I didn't check every day, but he has to understand that there will be weeks like this, and he has to recognize his responsibilities even if I am not there.

THERAPIST: Your week was stressful and it threw you off, and you might still be interested in getting back to the daily monitoring plan, to see how it could help Robert.

LEAH: Yes, I am still interested.

THERAPIST: Why?

LEAH: Because I made a commitment to trying these new strategies, even if I don't think they will work.

THERAPIST: You'd be up for trying again. That's very open-minded of you. What do you think it would take for you to be able to get in daily checks this week?

LEAH: The reality is that I'm not always home.

THERAPIST: You'd have to figure out a way to check even if you are not home.

LEAH: Maybe he can text me a picture of his planner when he gets home from school.

ROBERT: You want me to text you a picture?

LEAH: And then if you text it to me, when I get home after dinner, I'll let you have the video game controller. I can keep it in my car.

THERAPIST: So this is your idea for how to try again, and this time to reinforce the plan by finding a way that works for your busy schedule to check his planner. I get the sense that you are going to make it happen this week.

LEAH: I'm going to try.

Discussion: Progress Review

To remain grounded in the goals and values articulated by families in engagement module 2, each skill module includes a discussion of treatment goals—both progress and reasons for wanting to achieve these goals. Disclosures during this discussion can include parents' and teens' observations about themselves or about the other person. The purpose of holding these weekly discussions is to help the parent and teen maintain a clear vision of *why* changes are important to them and to make sure all small successes are celebrated during treatment—even during discouraging weeks.

Following is an excerpt from a progress review with Robert and Leah.

THERAPIST: Before we talk about a new skill for today, would you be willing to check in for a few minutes on how you each are doing on the goals you set for yourselves a few weeks ago?

LEAH: Sure.

THERAPIST: Leah, maybe we can start with you. What goals have you been working on?

LEAH: I've been working on finding ways to keep track of what Robert is doing even when I'm at work and also to be more strict with him when he doesn't do his part.

THERAPIST: You decided to spend our time together working out how to create some structure at home and oversee it. It's definitely a challenge because of

---

KEY POINT: Progress Review

Below are key topics that may be reviewed in a weekly progress review with the family.

- Ask the parent and teen to recall personal change goals made in engagement module 2.
- Ask the parent and teen to disclose anything that happened in support of these goals during the last week.
- Check whether families are continuing skills introduced in prior weeks.
- Elicit change talk from family members about the importance of treatment goals
- Affirm all parent and teen efforts—even if small.
- Reflect mobilizing change talk to elaborate on actions taken in support of goals.
- Elicit preparatory change talk about changes that have not yet begun.
- Link parent and teen actions to treatment goals and hopes for the future.

your work schedule, and I wonder what steps you've seen yourself take so far in support of these goals.

LEAH: Well, we've been making plans that give Robert an idea of what he is supposed to be doing.

THERAPIST: You've started giving him clear expectations, which is beginning to create a new structure at home.

LEAH: Right.

THERAPIST: And as we look forward to this upcoming week, what next steps are you considering to keep working on your goals?

LEAH: Well, we talked about having him text the picture, and then I've got to keep control of the video games.

THERAPIST: That plan would require you to take time out of your day to pay attention to whether he's texted you and also to remember to restrict access to the video games when necessary. On a scale from 0 to 10, with 0 being "not at all" and 10 being "very much," how confident are you that you will be able to try out these steps?

LEAH: I guess maybe a 6.

THERAPIST: You picked a 6. What made you pick that number and not, say, a 3?

LEAH: I guess I've made a commitment to trying out this plan. I'm just worried because it's honestly very challenging to add these little extra steps into my day.

THERAPIST: You worry that the little steps will be hard to keep on top of, and yet you really want to try out the plan this week.

LEAH: Yes, I do.

THERAPIST: Why are these goals important to you?

LEAH: I am sick of dealing with him. Nothing we've tried has worked. So I'm willing to trust that this could work, and I know that if we don't at least try it, we won't be able know for sure if the plan is bad or not.

THERAPIST: Even though you aren't confident these are the right ideas, you are willing to try them out as a learning experience. That says something about you as a mom—that you are willing to give anything a chance if it has a possibility of making home better for you and Robert.

Discussion: Introduce Skill

Skill introduction follows an EPE format (see Chapter 3 and Figure 6.3 on the next page). We see an example of skill introduction from a session with Kelley and Diane (see Chapter 4).

Step 1: Elicit from the family what they remember about relevant attention, EF, or motivation deficits. Ask how these deficits may impact the module's specific domain.

Step 2: Use EPE to discuss how the teen's cognitive deficits might lead to problem areas in the skill domain. This may include sharing scientific information about the teen's deficits.

Step 3: Introduce the idea that compensatory skills can help the teen overcome stated difficulties.

Step 4: Ask the family to share compensatory strategies that they have used in the past to help with the domain in question.

Step 5: Share the module's skill as a suggested compensatory strategy. Elicit the family's reaction to this skill and past experiences using it.

Step 6: Ask the teen how open he or she is to trying the skill during the next week.

Step 7: Encourage the teen to express perceived benefits and concerns with the strategy.

Step 8: Reflect change talk in favor of the approach, sidestep sustain talk against the approach, and seed ambivalence if the teen appears to be against trying the skill (see Chapter 4).

FIGURE 6.3. Steps for introducing skills using EPE.

THERAPIST: OK, well, then, to start out, let's talk about time management and planning for a second. Kelley, you and your mom both agreed that was an area of difficulty for you.

KELLEY: Mostly when something isn't due the next day. Like if I have a while until I know it's due, I'll procrastinate, and then it can be too late to get it done. That's my main problem.

DIANE: I think that she also has a problem slowing down and spending enough time on her work. A lot of times, she does it on the way to school or in the morning right before classes start. And I don't think she is doing her best work when she rushes through at the last minute like that.

THERAPIST: Problems with procrastinating, finding time to get things done, and having to rush when there isn't enough time—what you are describing is really common with a lot of families we work with.

KELLEY: Really?

THERAPIST: Sure. What do you remember about executive functioning? We talked about this a little in our first meeting.

KELLEY: I remember that it means sometimes you have trouble keeping your mind organized.

THERAPIST: Right. I wonder what kind of link, if any, you see between executive functioning difficulties you are experiencing and these time management problems?

KELLEY: I guess keeping my mind organized to plan out how to use time.

THERAPIST: And we've also been talking a little bit about how getting motivated can be challenging for you. How might that play into time management for you?

KELLEY: Even if I have a plan, it's hard to follow it if I really don't feel like doing something.

THERAPIST: So you see a link between time management and both the trouble keeping your brain organized and the trouble keeping yourself motivated.

KELLEY: Yeah.

THERAPIST: The good news is, we've been able to help a lot of kids who are struggling with time management find strategies that seem to make these problems get a little better.

KELLEY: Like what?

THERAPIST: Well, there are a lot of different things you can try, and only you will know which strategy makes the most sense for you. Would you be interested in hearing about some of them today?

KELLEY: Sure.

THERAPIST: The way a lot of people who struggle with time management describe it, starting homework without a plan can be like going on a road trip to a new place without a map or directions. What's your thought about that?

KELLEY: I get what you are saying, like before you go, you have to know where you are going.

THERAPIST: Without the map, you'd probably get there eventually, but you might be late because you have to stop to ask for directions or turn around a lot.

KELLEY: That makes sense.

THERAPIST: So one way to make a map before you get started is to create a list. What are either of your experiences with using lists to plan things out before you get started on them?

DIANE: I live off of lists at work. When you are a small business owner, you have to do a million things at once, so I have a notebook I use to keep track of what's going on and what I have to do next.

KELLEY: I don't think I've used a list.

DIANE: Yes, you have, I give you lists of chores to do all the time.

THERAPIST: Well, it's really up to you if you decide to use a strategy like that or not. Kelley, what are your thoughts on it?

KELLEY: I would try it. I'm not sure if I need that extra step of making a list, but I would try it if I have to.

THERAPIST: You are open to this idea of using lists to map out homework assignments ahead of time. How do you think it might help?

KELLEY: Well, I guess I could figure out what to do at the after-school program and what can wait until I come home.

DIANE: Finally, that is what I wanted to hear you say.

THERAPIST: Kelley, you think it could help you get on top of your work to make a plan ahead of time. What would it be like for you if that happened?

KELLEY: Well, I don't think it would actually benefit me in any way personally, but it might get my mom to leave me alone.

THERAPIST: Getting mom off your back would be a step in the right direction.

KELLEY: Yeah.

In-Session Exercise: Create Practice Plan

The therapist can explain that, to decide whether a skill is right for a teen, families typically practice for a week and then form an opinion. To decide the details of skill practice, the parent and the teen create a practice plan and then turn it into a contract.

Using the skill module worksheets, the family and the therapist can discuss adaptation of the weekly skill to the family's unique needs. The therapist can lead the teen and parent in a discussion that designates what needs to happen to prepare the teen for skill use (e.g., if there are supplies that must be obtained or actions that must be taken before starting the plan), how the teen will use the skill each day, and what the parent's role in reinforcing skill use will be.

In-Session Exercise: Introduce This Week's Skill Experiment ✪

Following completion of the practice plan, the therapist can lead the family to create a parent–teen contract that details (A) the teen's daily skill use, (B) a list of activities that must wait until after the skill is practiced, (C) what the parent will do to reinforce the contract, and (D) what the parent will do to ensure that the teen completes

---

KEY POINT: When Families Ask for Direct Advice

During practice planning, it is common for families to seek the advice of the therapist. In return, the therapist should emphasize parent and teen autonomy in knowing what will be best for their family. However, the therapist is free to use EPE to share ideas that have worked for other families in the past if this advice is solicited by the parent or teen. As part of this discussion, the therapist can ask the family how the ideas that worked for other families might fit with their situation. The therapist should refrain from using persuasion during these conversations.

responsibilities independently (for an example, see Worksheet 6.2). This contract is structured as outlined in engagement module 4 (see Chapter 5).

Home Exercise: Implement Weekly Skill Experiment

The therapist can review the details of the parent–teen contract. The parent and teen can be asked whether they are willing to follow the contract for 1 week. As a key element of the weekly skill experiment, the therapist should encourage the parent and teen to track how the practice plan went each day using the boxes at the bottom of the contract worksheet. The family can be encouraged to take notes on anything about the contract that they want to discuss at the upcoming session. The therapist can use the readiness ruler (see Chapter 4) during discussion of the home exercise to assess each family member's willingness to try the contract for a week, as well as his or her level of confidence in successfully carrying out their roles in the practice plan.

Skill Module 1: Writing Down Homework

Checklist for Skill Module 1

Materials

☐ Any device or notebook teen currently uses to record homework

Worksheets

☐ Worksheet 6.1. Writing Down Homework Practice Plan
☐ Worksheet 6.2. Writing Down Homework Contract

Case Example for Skill Module 1: Lisa and Miguel

Lisa is a single working mother who lives with her son Miguel, a seventh-grade student placed in small special education classes to address his disruptive classroom behavior. Prior to treatment, Lisa and Miguel's teachers reported that Miguel does not complete homework, frequently receives detentions for being disrespectful to teachers, and is often bullied by peers for being overweight. Fraught with a worry that Miguel will fail the school year, Lisa reports frequently completing Miguel's homework for him because he works very slowly through his work, often leaves his seat during homework, and complains that he does not understand his assignments. Lisa expressed a desire to hold Miguel accountable for behavior problems in school but typically resorts to lectures as a means of addressing his misbehavior.

Discussion: Review of Weekly Skill Experiment

Refer to "Structure of the Universal Skill Module" for instructions on how to conduct a review of the weekly skill experiment.

Discussion: Progress Review

Refer to "Structure of the Universal Skill Module" for instructions on how to conduct a progress review.

Discussion: Introduce Skill

Refer to "Structure of the Universal Skill Module" for instructions on how to conduct skill introduction. The central topic of this EPE-style discussion is how EF or attention deficits can lead to difficulties remembering homework. The key skill is writing down homework assignments to overcome difficulties remembering homework.

Therapeutic Progress

At the beginning of the session, Miguel insisted that he could remember homework assignments without resorting to writing them down, expressing displeasure at the idea of having to take the step of opening an agenda and writing down his assignments. Lisa expressed a concern that when Miguel becomes distracted in class, he often does not hear homework announcements. Both Lisa and Miguel agreed that using an agenda would be helpful—after all, Miguel had consistently used one in elementary school under the supervision of his special education teacher. His current teacher team had emphasized to Lisa that in middle school students are responsible for tracking their own assignments. As a result, she had given up on the planner as a reliable strategy for keeping track of Miguel's assignments. Despite their doubts, the two confirmed that they were open to trying out the skill of writing homework in a planner for 1 week—if only to observe what happened when Miguel attempted this practice without the assistance of a teacher.

In-Session Exercise: Create Practice Plan

Refer to "Structure of the Universal Skill Module" for instructions on how to create a practice plan with the family. Using Worksheet 6.1, the family and the therapist can create a practice plan for writing down homework. As part of this plan, the family must designate what type of notebook or device the teen will use to record homework, when he or she will do so, what he or she will write down if there is

---

KEY POINT: Why Is It So Hard to Remember Homework?

Teens with attention, EF, or motivation problems may display difficulties in the ability to pay attention to information being assigned, to accurately keep track of details (or steps) of an assignment, and to remember to complete tasks. When these skills are impaired, teens may have trouble remembering homework assignments without compensatory skills (such as a written system for keeping track of assignments).

> **KEY POINT: Teacher Involvement in Writing Down Homework**
>
> When students are forgetful, parents may be unsure whether assignments written in a daily agenda are correct or complete. Moreover, when students fail to record homework in a class, it may be unclear whether no homework was assigned or whether the student forgot to record it.
>
> A logical solution to this problem is to ask teachers to verify the accuracy of the student's planner—usually by placing their initials next to the recorded assignment. Typically, secondary school teachers will agree to do so if the student approaches them after class and asks them to sign his or her planner. However, secondary school teachers are very busy between classes and rarely will be able to approach the student for verification themselves.
>
> In general, teacher verification is helpful when the student has a history of incorrectly recording homework assignments. Many students do not need to have these supports in place to accurately implement this skill. Some families find it helpful to engage teachers only when the student indicates that there is no homework.

no homework (to protect against being accused of forgetting), when the parent will check to see if the assignments were written down, and whether the teacher should be involved in checking recorded homework for accuracy.

Therapeutic Progress

While creating a plan for agenda use, Lisa indicated that Miguel owned a planner, which was given to him by the school at the beginning of the school year. Miguel stated that he knew where the planner was and would retrieve it from his room upon returning home from the therapy session. He also volunteered to write his homework in the planner at the end of each class. When discussing what to do when no homework was assigned by the teacher, Miguel indicated that he would leave his agenda blank. With permission, the therapist offered a suggestion that had worked for a lot of families in the past—namely, that writing either "no homework" or "none" might be a way of communicating to his mother that he had not simply forgotten to write down homework but that none had been assigned. Returning again to the issue of teacher involvement in the agenda intervention, the therapist offered another piece of advice: Families often see success when teens approach the teacher independently to ask him or her to write his or her initials in the planner (rather than expecting the teacher to proactively verify what the teen writes). Although Lisa agreed that this might be a useful approach, she reiterated that she wanted to see what would happen if Miguel independently managed his homework agenda for the next week.

In-Session Exercise: Introduce This Week's Skill Experiment ✪

Refer to "Structure of the Universal Skill Module" for instructions on how to introduce a weekly skill experiment. Worksheet 6.2 is a contract template for skill module 1.

In a group setting, it may be appropriate to cover more than one skill module in a single session. All group sessions begin with a joint home activity review from the last session.

Parent Content: Using the subgroup discussion format, parents can be prompted to discuss their past experiences recording homework. Worksheet 6.1 can be used to facilitate discussion of possibilities for planner use.

Teen Content: Teens can also discuss the benefits of using a planner and their past experiences using this skill. The therapist can complete Worksheet 6.1 with teens.

Collaborative Content ○: Parents and teens can discuss the contents of Worksheet 6.1 and can complete Worksheet 6.2, which details a contract for planner use.

FIGURE 6.4. Delivering skill module 1 as a group.

Home Exercise: Implement Weekly Skill Experiment

The family should follow the contract detailed on Worksheet 6.2 for 1 week.

Skill Module 2: Making a Homework Plan

Checklist for Skill Module 2

Materials

☐ None

Worksheets

☐ Worksheet 6.3. Homework Practice Plan
☐ Worksheet 6.4. Homework Contract

Case Example for Skill Module 2: Sheryl and Daniel

Daniel is an 11-year-old boy who lives with his adoptive parents and three siblings. His mother, Sheryl, presented for treatment with concerns that Daniel displayed difficulty organizing his school belongings, was often unsure of what was assigned for homework, and lacked focus during homework time. She also complained that her own attention difficulties interfere with her ability to create consistent structure at home. Daniel appeared implicitly respectful to his mother, who in turn reflected

KEY POINT: Why Is It So Hard to Focus during Homework?

Teens with attention, EF, or motivation problems may display difficulties in tuning out distractions, completing work when a task is hard or boring, and sustaining attention over time. Distractions during homework time often relate specifically to motivation problems, which can lead teens to seek relief from boring and uncomfortably aversive activities by fixing attention on more interesting stimuli (e.g., cell phones, electronics). Teens who struggle with these deficits may have trouble independently managing their homework.

patience and kindness when interacting with her son. Though he was the highest functioning of his siblings, Daniel struggled in a household that was a chaotic combination of four youth with behavioral or developmental concerns and a parent who, although devoted and compassionate, struggled to create structure and consistency due to her own attention problems.

Review of Weekly Skill Experiment

Refer to "Structure of the Universal Skill Module" for instructions on how to conduct a review of the weekly skill experiment.

Progress Review

Refer to "Structure of the Universal Skill Module" for instructions on how to conduct a progress review.

Discussion: Introduce Skill

Refer to "Structure of the Universal Skill Module" for instructions on how to conduct skill introduction. The central topic of this EPE-style discussion can be how EF, motivation, or attention deficits can interfere with staying focused during homework time. The key skill is coming up with a strategic plan that communicates a consistent homework routine each day. This routine includes details about where and when homework will be done and how to remove and resist distractions in the homework environment.

Therapeutic Progress

When discussing why students may struggle to stay on-task during homework, Daniel offered that boredom is the primary reason why he has difficulty completing work efficiently. The therapist affirmed Daniel's struggle to stay motivated when assignments seem boring and asked what strategies he had tried to increase on-task behavior after school. Sheryl quickly volunteered that she had been considering removing electronics until after Daniel showed proof that he completed his homework. Daniel immediately interrupted to state that his sister with special needs was actually the biggest distraction during homework time—not his electronics. Though Sheryl and Daniel seemed eager to solve the problem of distractions at home during this discussion about the nature of homework problems, the therapist asked the pair if they would be delay problem solving until later in the session, and they obliged.

In-Session Exercise: Create Practice Plan

Refer to "Structure of the Universal Skill Module" for instructions on how to create a practice plan with the family. Using Worksheet 6.3, the family and the therapist can create a practice plan for homework time. As part of this plan, the family can designate how long the teen should spend on homework, what distractions must be removed from the homework environment, the parent's current and desired role in homework completion, and any other challenges that make homework time difficult for families.

Therapeutic Progress

In sharing the current state of homework time, Daniel explained that he typically spends 3 hours on homework. Sheryl elaborated that although Daniel spends about 3 hours seated in front of his homework, he is probably only actively completing homework for about 1 hour. Throughout the conversation, Daniel continued to bring up his concern about his sister's distracting behaviors. When expanding on this concern, Sheryl and Daniel listed additional distractions—the blender, the vacuum cleaner—ultimately realizing that all loud noises are highly distracting to Daniel when he tries to complete his schoolwork. Sheryl expressed a desire to find a quieter location for Daniel to complete homework but was unsure of how she would monitor his progress if she removed him from the central area of the house. She added that she believed Daniel also experiences distractions in his own mind, a problem she felt only his medication would solve—medication that wears off after 3:00 P.M. The therapist asked what Sheryl thought she could do to support her own goal of increasing structure and consistency at home, and she stated that she would like to create a planned homework routine for Daniel, as well as her other three children.

In-Session Exercise: Introduce This Week's Skill Experiment ✪

Refer to "Structure of the Universal Skill Module" for instructions on how to introduce a weekly skill experiment. Worksheet 6.4 is a contract template for skill module 2.

Therapeutic Progress

During contract negotiation, Daniel says that he will complete homework Monday through Friday afternoons. Sheryl stops to ask Daniel whether he is comfortable completing weekend homework on Fridays rather than waiting until Sunday. Stating that he would like to enjoy his weekend without worrying about homework, Daniel confirms that he would like to designate Friday as a homework day. The therapist asks the family to consider what they will do if Daniel comes home without any assigned homework. Sheryl and Daniel decide that Daniel will study for an upcoming test for an hour if he does not have any homework. They agree that he will begin homework by 4:30 each day and may not move on to enjoyable activities until he shows his completed work to his mother. Sheryl decided that she would ask Daniel to relinquish his cell phone when he returns from school until homework is completed but hesitates when considering whether to restrict his computer use after school.

KEY POINT: *Homework Contract Details*

The details of the homework contract will vary by family. Some considerations may be useful to discuss.

Days of the week. Clear expectations should be made about on which days of the week homework will be done. If weekend homework is assigned, the family should create a structured plan for which day of the week these assignments will be completed. In addition, if the adolescent says he or she has no homework on a homework day (e.g., Tuesday), the family should discuss whether additional studying or project work should occur anyway, to keep a consistent homework routine.

Start and stop time. When a family's afternoon routine is predictable and consistent, it may be helpful to set an exact time (e.g., 4:00 P.M.) by which the teen must start homework. When schedules vary throughout the week, some families may choose to designate an amount of time between arriving home and starting homework (e.g., 30 minutes). Stop time typically occurs when the adolescent demonstrates proof that work is complete. However, in some cases, families may choose to designate a specific time for stopping homework. This strategy may be appropriate when an adolescent chooses to perseverate on work or if a privilege is made contingent upon completing work by a certain time each night.

Distraction-free environment. No environment is completely distraction free; however, efforts to reduce distractions can greatly improve homework time. These efforts include removing all access to electronics until homework is complete, creating a quiet homework space, and separating teens from family members who may interrupt homework. Teens may insist that they need their devices to complete certain homework assignments. In this case, the family may decide to allow supervised access to devices only when the teen is actively working on assignments that require their use. Finally, when quiet homework spaces are located away from the parent, efforts can be made to create accountability for homework completion by asking the teen to show proof of completed work before allowing participation in fun activities.

Homework rules. Families may designate homework rules that specify competing activities that the adolescent may not enjoy until after homework is complete. Rules may also indicate the number of breaks the adolescent may take, how these breaks may be earned, and whether and when the adolescent can ask the parent for help. Careful consideration of the adolescent's presenting homework problems may lead to family-specific homework rules.

Parent's role. In describing the parent's role in homework time, it is important to designate both what the parent will do and what the parent will *not* do. Appropriate accountability for following the homework contract requires monitoring. However, building independent skill use requires parents to withhold reminders, redirection, and assistance in favor of collaborative planning, expectation setting, and accountability for not following the contract.

Enjoyable activities. The parent and teen should consider two separate ways to earn enjoyable activities—one for completing work and another for following the rules of the contract. This strategy allows a teen to break a contract rule (and experience a consequence) and still find motivation to continue completing homework (because a different consequence is associated with completion, regardless of rule breaking). For example, an enjoyable activity may be offered as soon as homework is complete. However, if the teen is caught breaking a rule (e.g., looking at social media before homework is complete), he or she may have to perform a chore after homework time and before the enjoyable activity is allowed.

In a group setting, it may be appropriate to cover more than one skill module in a single session. All group sessions begin with a joint home activity review from the last session.

Parent Content: Using the subgroup discussion format, parents can be prompted to discuss their current challenges during homework time and current involvement in homework. Worksheet 6.3 can be used to facilitate discussion of current homework time issues.

Teen Content: Teens can also discuss challenges they experience during homework time. The therapist can complete Worksheet 6.3 with teens to expand upon the details of homework difficulties.

Collaborative Content ♺: Parents and teens can discuss the contents of Worksheet 6.3 and can complete Worksheet 6.4, negotiating a homework contract.

FIGURE 6.5. Delivering skill module 2 in a group.

Daniel openly shared that he often needs his computer to complete his homework but that he struggles to resist the temptation to watch online videos when he wants a break from work. Ultimately, the pair decide to require Daniel to complete noncomputer homework first—in his mother's bedroom, which was decidedly the quietest location in the house. Once it was time for computer homework, he would bring the laptop into the kitchen so that Sheryl could keep an eye on his use. Though both felt the contract was not perfect, they agreed that it represented a good step in the right direction and conceded that a perfect solution to their dilemma may not exist.

Home Exercise: Implement Weekly Skill Experiment

The family should follow the contract detailed on Worksheet 6.2 for one week.

Skill Module 3: Organization Checkups

Checklist for Skill Module 3

Materials

☐ Teen book bag, binders, folders, and other academic materials

Worksheets

☐ Worksheet 6.5 Guide to Staying Organized
☐ Worksheet 6.6. Sample Organization Checkup Practice Plan
☐ Worksheet 6.7. Organization Checkup Practice Plan
☐ Worksheet 6.8. Organization Contract

Case Example for Skill Module 3: Kate and Richard

Kate is a recently divorced mother of two who just received full custody of her children. Her son, Richard, is a gifted and talented student in ninth grade at a local public school. Kate reports that Richard has a very poorly organized bedroom and backpack. As such, he frequently cannot find and turn in completed assignments. She also indicated that she frequently holds discussions with Richard about his disorganization but has never taken steps to remediate these difficulties because she believes he is old enough to manage his own belongings. She reports continued stress from her divorce and a desire for Richard to take on increased responsibilities in the home setting given that he is now, in her own words, the "new man of the house." Kate also mentions that Richard experiences difficulty falling asleep at night, which sometimes means that he cannot wake for school on time in the morning. She believes Richard's sleep problems are a contributor to his disorganization. After waking up late, he often rushes out the door in the morning, leaving no time to neaten his room and backpack. He requires a nap after school to prepare for homework, also leaving no time to clean his room and book bag after school.

Review of Weekly Skill Experiment

Refer to "Structure of the Universal Skill Module" for instructions on how to conduct a review of the weekly skill experiment.

Progress Review

Refer to "Structure of the Universal Skill Module" for instructions on how to conduct a progress review.

Discussion: Introduce Skill

Refer to "Structure of the Universal Skill Module" for instructions on how to conduct skill introduction. The central topic of this EPE-style discussion can be how EF or attention deficits can lead to difficulties keeping belongings organized. The key skill is creating a system for organizing belongings and performing regular checks of this system that include corrections when the teen deviates from the system.

As part of this discussion, the therapist can emphasize that successful skill use includes both setting up an initial system *and* performing regular organization checkups.

KEY POINT: What Leads to Disorganization?

Teens with attention, EF, or motivation problems may display difficulties keeping track of belongings, noticing when belongings become disorganized, and staying motivated to keep belongings neat. When these skills are impaired, teens may have trouble keeping an organized book bag, which may lead to lost or damaged schoolwork.

> **KEY POINT: Checkups versus Interference**
>
> A commonly reported source of parental overinvolvement in academics is micromanagement of the adolescent's book bag and school materials. Some parents regularly organize and sort through the teen's belongings in an attempt to keep them organized. Although this strategy leads to an organized backpack, it does not teach the teen to organize him- or herself. The organization checkup system requires the teen to manage his or her own belongings. The parent conducts checkups and sends the adolescent to correct his or her own disorganization before being allowed to enjoy other activities.

Therapeutic Progress

When discussing what they already know about organization difficulties, Richard states that he knows some people are more naturally organized than others but believes that anyone can be organized if they learn the right skills. Kate discloses that when she was younger, she also struggled to stay organized but that she now stays on top of her life by using an agenda and lists—skills she hopes her son will also develop. Kate reiterates that she sees her son as very bright, but scattered. Richard agrees and says that he is able to stay organized at the beginning of each school year but slowly tends toward disorganization as months pass. Kate relates her tendency to also become disorganized when she fails to pause and reset certain aspects of her life. The therapist linked this experience to the idea of creating periodic checkups to reorganize.

In-Session Exercise: Create Practice Plan

Refer to "Structure of the Universal Skill Module" for instructions on how to create a practice plan with the family. Using Worksheet 6.5, the family and the therapist can create a plan for reorganizing a messy book bag to prepare it for its first checkup. This process may include cleaning out unnecessary belongings, deciding on an organization system, documenting the system on a checklist, and scheduling the regular checks.

To begin this process, the therapist can spend time in session working with the parent and the teen to clean out the teen's book bag, beginning the reorganization process. It may be necessary to obtain additional supplies to complete initial organization of the book bag, and the parent and teen may identify these supplies and discuss how they will be obtained.

Next, the therapist can refer to Worksheets 6.6 and 6.7 to provide an example of an organization practice plan that a previous client family used to document the criteria for an organized book bag. The family can refer to this example as they work with the clinician to create their own organization practice plan.

KEY POINT: *Choosing Checkup Criteria*

The first step of the organization checkup is determining organization criteria. Possible criteria are outlined here.

Where should papers be? Unruly papers are the chief culprit when a homework assignment is lost. Many families choose an overarching criterion stating that all papers must be stored securely in appropriate designated locations. It is also useful to provide a separate folder or binder for each class so that papers do not intermix.

Choosing a storage system. Adolescents may choose to store papers in folders, separate binders, or a single binder with separate sections for each class. Binders may contain hole-punched folders or dividers for each class. In designing a storage system, the principle of simplicity can be particularly helpful to adolescents with attention and EF deficits. Therefore, the fewer parts to the system, the easier it often is for the adolescent to keep track of his or her belongings.

Permissible contents. The parent and teen should carefully discuss contents that may and may not be in the backpack. Nonacademic contents can create clutter that exacerbates organization problems.

Homework storage. A homework storage plan is a strategic way to reduce lost homework assignments. One suggestion that typically serves families very well is to have a separate homework folder that is only used to carry assignments that have yet to be turned in. Use of a homework folder increases the adolescent's ability to find homework when the teacher asks for it.

Ideas for sample organization criteria can be found on Worksheet 6.6.

Therapeutic Progress

Kate and Richard decided to brainstorm organization criteria. This process started with what turned out to be a very clear visual depiction of his current difficulties. When prompted by the therapist, Richard pulled out his green canvas backpack, tugging the snagged zipper back and forth until it released, spilling its contents on the table. He grasped two tattered spiral notebooks and set them next to a 2-inch red binder piped with residual graphite from months of friction against broken pencils. Left in his bag was mass of dog-eared papers, a flattened pair of gym socks, and various writing utensils—damaged from maltreatment and dripping in sticky blue ink. He looked sheepishly at his mother and therapist and narrated the scene in front of them. Richard disclosed that he currently used one notebook for his morning classes and one for his afternoon classes and that he liked his current system. During this conversation, Kate discovered that Richard had lost his Spanish workbook and found an important permission form crumpled at the bottom of his bag. These experiences led them to design a checklist for Richard that required him to have no loose papers in his bag; all books, notebooks, and folders present; and a designated folder with one pocket for yet-to-be-completed homework assignments and another for papers that needed to be given to his mother. Richard also expressed a concern that he often had loose papers because the teacher distributed worksheets without holes in them and his current binder had no pockets. As a result, Kate agreed to purchase plastic pocketed dividers to place in his school binder—one for each class. They also designated the front pocket of his backpack for pens and pencils.

In-Session Exercise: Introduce Weekly Skill Experiment ⊗

Refer to "Structure of the Universal Skill Module" for instructions on how to introduce a weekly skill experiment. Worksheet 6.8 is a contract template for skill module 3.

Therapeutic Progress

Considering the severity of Richard's disorganization, Kate suggested that they perform a checkup twice a week, possibly moving to once a week once Richard showed progress. They decided to hold checkups on Sunday and Wednesday, the beginning and middle of the week. Richard insisted that he could meet all criteria at each checkup and agreed to immediately correct any unmet criteria. When discussing which enjoyable activities must wait until Richard organized his book bag, he asked for 10 dollars each time he successful passed the inspection. Kate expressed concerns about the message communicated by paying her son to be organized. Ultimately, the two decided that Richard would earn a point for each inspection he passed and that, after 10 points, he would be able to go to the hobby store for a new model airplane. Kate decided that prior to each checkup, she would give Richard a 5-minute warning. She also decided to set a reminder in her smartphone to ensure that she remembered to perform the check.

Home Exercise: Implement Organization Inspection

The family should follow the contract detailed on Worksheet 6.8 for 1 week.

KEY POINT: How to Contract When Checkups Are Not Done Daily

Typically, it is not necessary for parents and teens to perform organization checkups on a daily basis. It can become complicated to connect a nondaily responsibility to a daily privilege. Instead, the family may consider using a point system toward a long-term enjoyable activity (one that does not occur on a regular basis). For example, a teen who occasionally enjoys going to the movies with friends can wait to do so until he or she has passed 10 organization inspections. The concept of putting responsibilities first remains the same; in this case the earned activity is one the teen would typically enjoy on an intermittent basis, not a new reward. As part of this contract, the parent must agree to allow access to the enjoyable activity only when the teen has met the criteria for earning it.

In a group setting, it may be appropriate to cover more than one skill module in a single session. All group sessions begin with a joint home activity review from the last session.

Parent Content: Using the subgroup discussion format, parents can be prompted to discuss their current challenges with teens' organization and current involvement in keeping their teens organized. Next, parents can draft sample organization inspection criteria.

Teen Content: Teens can also discuss challenges they experience with organization. As part of this process they can discuss potential organization inspection criteria and their thoughts on implementing an inspection intervention.

Collaborative Content ✪: Parents and teens can compare their inspection criteria on **Worksheet 20** and can finalize a list. The parent and teen can negotiate a plan for inspecting backpack organization using Worksheet 6.8.

FIGURE 6.6. Delivering skill module 3 in a group.

Skill Module 4: Time Management Strategies

Checklist for Skill Module 4

Materials

☐ List of teen's assigned homework (e.g., daily planner or device)

Worksheets

☐ Worksheet 6.9. How to Break Down Tasks to Get Started

☐ Worksheet 6.10. Sample Homework List

☐ Worksheet 6.11. Time Management Contract

Case Example for Skill Module 4: Rita and Rose

Rita is a young mother who owns and operates a small local coffee shop. Her 16-year-old daughter, Rose, is a competitive swimmer who is placed in regular classes at a local high school. In Sessions 1 and 2, Rita expressed concerns that Rose rushes through her homework and often fails to turn in assignments. During the first quarter of the academic year, Rose received an F in her math class for failing to complete daily online learning modules. Rose states that the C's she earns are sufficient, complaining instead that her mother is constantly nagging her about homework. Rose also indicates a concern that her mother does not let her spend enough time with her friends and that she wants to start driving but that her mother won't take her to get her license.

Review of Weekly Skill Experiment

Refer to "Structure of the Universal Skill Module" for instructions on how to conduct a review of the weekly skill experiment.

Progress Review

Refer to "Structure of the Universal Skill Module" for instructions on how to conduct a progress review.

Discussion: Introduce Skill

Refer to "Structure of the Universal Skill Module" for instructions on how to conduct skill introduction. The central topic of this EPE-style discussion can be how EF, motivation, or attention deficits can lead to difficulties with time management. Two components of time management can be discussed in this session: difficulties getting started on work and trouble making and carrying out a plan. An excellent analogy for this latter skill deficit is trying to go on a road trip without a map. The two skills that are included in this module are breaking tasks into small components to overcome motivation problems and making lists to help with planning.

Therapeutic Progress

Rita expressed eagerness to discuss time management with her daughter. Rose said that when she knows an assignment is not due right away, she procrastinates until it is often too late to complete the assignment carefully and by deadline. Rita confirmed that Rose often rushes through assignments and leaves them until the last minute, attempting to complete them on the way to school or in between classes. Rose complained that she returns home from swim practice late and that by the time she begins homework her brain is too tired to focus on schoolwork. She conceded that getting up early in the morning to do her homework might help, since her mind is tired after swim practice. The therapist introduces the idea of using a list to plan before starting homework. Rita confirms that she often uses this technique in her business—beginning her day with a cup of coffee and a to-do list. The two agreed that this strategy would likely be helpful for Rose, allowing her to decide the appropriate time to fit each homework assignment into her busy schedule. During this conversation, the therapist provided reflections to Rose that highlighted a salient potential benefit of using the list strategy—namely, that her mother might reduce reminders and complaints about her homework completion.

> **KEY POINT: Where Do Time Management Problems Come From?**
>
> Teens with attention, EF, or motivation problems may display difficulties in their ability to estimate how much time is required for a given task, to accurately judge the passage of time, and to remember long-term assignments. They may also struggle to find motivation to begin tasks when they perceive them as difficult or boring. When these skills are impaired, teens may have trouble staying on top of long-term assignments and homework completion without compensatory skills.

In-Session Exercise: Create Practice Plan

Refer to "Structure of the Universal Skill Module" for instructions on how to create a practice plan with the family. Using Worksheet 6.9, the therapist can introduce the strategy of breaking tasks into smaller and smaller parts when it feels hard to get started on work. As part of this worksheet, the therapist can guide the parent and teen to consider the example and then try the strategy out on their own.

Using Worksheet 6.10, the family and the therapist can discuss how to use a list to plan out homework time. The therapist can guide the teen and parent in a demonstration of how to create a list for homework using the teen's homework assignments for that night. The categories on the sample list include long-term projects, online learning, reading, and studying, as well as nightly homework assignments. The therapist can prompt the teen to record all upcoming assignments in each category.

KEY POINT: How to Prioritize

Prioritization is an active process by which the teen reviews what needs to be done and how much time each task will take and decides when and in what order to complete tasks. Prioritization encourages teens' strategic decision making. When prioritizing, the teen might consider the following questions.

Urgency. Are there assignments that are due before others? Are there certain assignments that are highly weighted and would be most problematic if the teen could not get through everything on the list?

Overcoming motivation problems. Some individuals report that one way to overcome motivation problems is to start with smaller and easier tasks. Beginning with tasks that are less hard or boring can allow the teen get started on work more easily. Many times, getting started is the hardest part of a homework struggle. As noted, breaking tasks into small and manageable pieces is one way of reducing the perception that homework is hard or boring, facilitating the process of getting started.

Accurately estimating task duration. Evidence suggests that teens with attention or EF problems often misjudge the passage of time. Taking an extra step to consider how long a task will take can help the teen with planning. When estimating task duration, the teen should consider how long the task has taken in the past and offer a realistic estimate of its duration. When the teen misjudges, it is helpful for him or her to notice the actual task duration to correct future estimates.

Choosing when to work on homework. Many teens juggle extracurricular activities, transit, and home responsibilities after school. Though a stable homework time should be designated in the after-school routine (see skill module 2), it may be appropriate to capitalize on idle time to get a head start on homework. For example, shorter or easier tasks may be well suited for completion on the bus, when waiting for an after-school activity to begin, or during a free period at school.

Remembering long-term projects and upcoming tests. One of the greatest challenges for a teen with EF deficits is carrying out a long-term project or staggering study time for a test. Prioritization also includes noticing upcoming tests and projects and designating time to complete these tasks.

The second step to completing the homework to-do list is for the teen to esti-mate how long it will take to complete each item. Once this is done, the teen can discuss prioritization of tasks, numbering them to represent the order in which he or she decides to complete them. This is the process of prioritizing, and it should be carefully discussed with the teen. The teen can also be guided to make strategic deci-sions about when to complete each assignment (e.g., between school and practice, after dinner, in the morning, during a free period).

Finally, the therapist can instruct the teen to initial the list when a task is com-plete. As part of this conversation, the therapist and family members should discuss the parent's role in supporting list use. This may include having the parent help the teen make the list, having the teen show an independently completed list to the par-ent prior to homework, or waiting until after homework time to show all completed assignments to the parent. If a high level of monitoring seems appropriate for a particular adolescent, the parent may check the teen's work after each assignment.

Therapeutic Progress

When trying the list strategy, Rose consulted her planner and spent a minute writing down assignments that were due the next day. She paused before the test category and looked up at her mother and the therapist, expressing a concern that her teach-ers did not announce test dates until a few days before an exam, making it hard for her to study ahead of time. Rita asked Rose if she would be willing to study for a test even if she did not yet know the date of it, and Rose agreed. With respect to long-term projects, Rose disclosed an upcoming English essay but complained that she did not want to start it until the weekend. The therapist emphasized that Rose could make choices about whether and how much time to spend on each assignment on the list—even choosing to defer an assignment to another night. Given her busy sched-ule, Rose realized that time management decisions about long-term assignments must consider the entire week's outlook. Using the strategy of breaking tasks into smaller steps, Rose broke her essay into specific steps. In estimating how much time would be needed to complete these steps, she designated blocks of time to devote to her essay each night for the next few days.

Rita and Rose discussed giving priority to assignments that were worth a high percentage of Rose's grade—given the realistic risk that she might not always have time to complete all assignments with her busy schedule. During this conversation, Rose decided to get up early in the morning to spend a couple of hours on the most important daily assignments, to dedicate more time on the weekends to long-term projects, and to take advantage of breaks between activities to complete smaller daily assignments.

In a group setting, it may be appropriate to cover more than one skill module in a single session.

All group sessions begin with a joint home activity review from the last session.

Parent Content: Using the subgroup discussion format, parents can be prompted to discuss the concepts of prioritization and planning. As part of this discussion, the therapist can introduce Worksheet 6.10 and elicit parent impressions of the tool. The parents can discuss their potential role in supporting the teen to use this worksheet.

Teen Content: Teens can also discuss the concepts of planning and prioritizing. Worksheet 6.10 can be introduced and the teens can share their impressions of the tool. The therapist can guide teens to complete a planning and prioritization sheet for the evening.

Collaborative Content ✪: Teens can share their completed Worksheet 6.9 with parents, walking parents through their prioritization process. The parents and teens can use Worksheet 6.10 to negotiate a home contract for the homework to-do list and Worksheet 6.11 to fill out a time management contract.

FIGURE 6.7. Delivering skill module 4 in a group.

In-Session Exercise: Introduce This Week's Skill Experiment ✪

Refer to "Structure of the Universal Skill Module" for instructions on how to introduce a weekly skill experiment. Worksheet 6.11 is a contract template for skill module 4.

Therapeutic Progress

Rita and Rose decide to use the homework list for the next 4 school days. They decide to complete the list when they sit down together for dinner, right after Rose's swim practice. Rita expressed a desire to monitor whether Rose capitalizes on her free period at school—mentioning that it is an optimal time for her to complete homework assignments for her afternoon classes. They consider having Rose take a picture of work that she completes during her free period and texting this picture to Rita. Ultimately, they decide they can resort to that level of monitoring if necessary but that for the next 4 days Rose will show her mother what she plans to do in her free period and will text her each day to let her know what she actually was able to accomplish. During the contract, Rita and Rose indicated that all of Rose's enjoyable activities occur on the weekend, given her busy schedule during the week. As a result, Rita and Rose agreed that for appropriately practicing the list each day of the week, Rose would be allowed to go out with her friends on Saturday night.

Home Exercise: Implement Weekly Skill Experiment

The family should follow the contract detailed on Worksheet 6.11 for one week.

Skill Module 5: Study Skills

Checklist for Skill Module 5

Materials

☐ Blank note cards

Worksheets

☐ Worksheet 6.12. Active Studying

☐ Worksheet 6.13. Flash Cards

☐ Worksheet 6.14. Fake Word Activity: Flash Cards

☐ Worksheet 6.15. Notes from Text

☐ Worksheet 6.16. Study Plan

Case Example for Skill Module 5: Maxine and Edwin

Edwin is a 17-year-old 12th-grade student who attends advanced classes at a private high school. He is actively involved in speech and debate, student government, and cross country. His mother, Maxine, reports that despite being very bright, Edwin's test performance is inconsistent due to inadequate test preparation. She voiced a concern that Edwin will need to improve his study skills to be successful in college. She reports that although she used to be actively involved in Edwin's homework activities, she decided to end all involvement this year to prepare for his transition to college. Edwin reports that school performance and college are important to him but that he struggles to find motivation to study.

Review of Weekly Skill Experiment

Refer to "Structure of the Universal Skill Module" for instructions on how to conduct a review of the weekly skill experiment.

Progress Review

Refer to "Structure of the Universal Skill Module" for instructions on how to conduct a progress review.

Discussion: Introduce Skill

Refer to "Structure of the Universal Skill Module" for instructions on how to conduct skill introduction. The central topic of this EPE-style discussion can be how EF, motivation, or attention deficits can lead to difficulties succeeding on tests. The key skills are scheduling designated study sessions in preparation for a test and using active studying strategies during these sessions. Active studying includes a range of study techniques that require the teen to interact with and manipulate the material,

KEY POINT: Why Is Test Preparation So Hard?

Teens with attention, EF, or motivation problems may display difficulties in the ability to attend to and encode information, store it, and recall it when it is later needed. When these skills are impaired, teens may have trouble recalling information during a test. In addition, difficulties with time management, planning, and motivation often mean that adolescents do not set aside enough time to study for tests.

rather than passive reading or highlighting material. During this discussion, the therapist can refer to Worksheet 6.12, which provides examples of active and passive studying.

Therapeutic Progress

Edwin begins the discussion of study skills by describing the challenge of knowing he should study, pulling out his books, and not being able to force himself to open them. He indicates that when he attempts to study, he often reads material over and over again while his mind finds itself elsewhere. He expresses a genuine worry that he will not be able to complete college due to his difficulties preparing for tests. Edwin confesses that he has been considering medication as an option to help him focus while studying. However, he is somewhat uncomfortable taking medication due to past negative experiences. The therapist introduces the concept of active studying, asking Edwin whether he thinks such a strategy could help him overcome his studying difficulties. Edwin expresses openness to hearing about the techniques, acknowledging that his most successful attempts at study have involved taking notes on his course handouts and textbooks.

In-Session Exercise: Create Practice Plan

Refer to "Structure of the Universal Skill Module" for instructions on how to create a practice plan with the family. The therapist can introduce two active study skills that are particularly effective for teens with attention, EF, and motivation problems. One skill is flash cards, and the other is taking notes from reading materials. Though many youth have previously utilized flash cards to study, this tool can be used in several different ways—some effective and some ineffective. Referring to Worksheet 6.13, the therapist can discuss with the family the keys to effective flash card use.

The therapist, parent, and teen can complete the pseudo-word activity on Worksheet 6.14 as a way to practice and model effective flash card use. During this activity, the teen creates, studies, and demonstrates mastery of five pseudo-words using the active studying process (see Worksheet 6.12). With the teen's permission, the therapist can offer feedback on his or her performance throughout this task. After completing this activity, the therapist should discuss with the parent and teen their impressions of the active studying process applied to flash cards.

KEY POINT: Effective Use of Flash Cards

Many individuals use flash cards ineffectively. Effective flash card use for teens includes the following elements:

- The teen (not the parent or a tutor) should make the flash cards. Creating flash cards is an important part of the active studying process, exposing the brain to material.
- The front of the flash card should contain only one word or main idea.
- The back of the flash card should contain a bite-size piece of information—usually limited to four words.
- The teen should study flash cards independently to promote self-guided studying.
- The teen can go through the stack of flash cards to quiz him- or herself by placing in one pile correct cards and in one pile incorrect cards.
- The teen can continue to quiz him- or herself until all incorrect cards arrive in the correct pile.
- Mastery is reached when the stack can be gone through in 3 seconds per card or less (i.e., a stack of 20 cards can be recited in 60 seconds).
- The parent's role may be to quiz the adolescent *after* the adolescent claims mastery. This is different from quizzing the adolescent as he or she builds mastery. If the adolescent cannot yet recite the cards quickly, the parent should send him or her back to study longer.

The second active studying skill that the therapist can introduce is taking notes from readings. Creating reading notes involves pausing after each paragraph to jot down notes on important points.

Referring to Worksheet 6.15, the therapist can lead the teen through a reading notes activity in which the teen is asked to read a brief paragraph and to identify the main topic and supporting details that might show up on a test later. With the teen's permission, the therapist can offer corrective feedback during this task and ask the teen's impressions after task completion. See Figure 6.8 for sample flash cards and reading notes.

KEY POINT: Reading Notes

Reading educational material can be one of the most challenging tasks for teens with attention, EF, and motivation problems; internal distractions may lead the teen to think about irrelevant information when scanning the page. As a result, the material often is not retained, and this can be most problematic when it will later appear on a test. Key points for creating reading notes are:

- The teen should pause after each paragraph to consider what information might be most important.
- The teen should write down the main topic of the paragraph to help organize notes.
- Underneath the main topic, the teen should write down any important details that might later appear on a test.
- Once a set of reading notes is complete, they can later be converted into flash cards to enhance mastery of material.

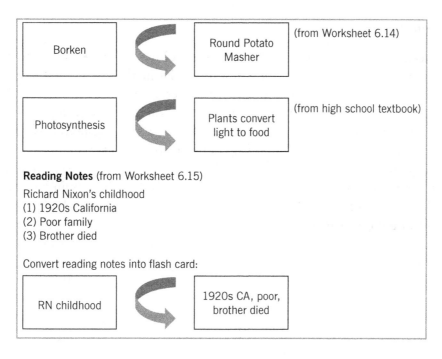

FIGURE 6.8. Sample flash cards and reading notes.

Therapeutic Progress

Edwin expressed an opinion that flash cards were for younger students, and the therapist revealed that college students often use the technique to prepare for exams. Though initially Edwin was surprised at this detail, he increased his openness to trying flash cards upon hearing this. Edwin and the therapist completed the flash card activity and discussed how the techniques could be used to remember facts—an ability Edwin was interested in improving. Following the flash card activity, the therapist reviewed the reading notes skill, one that Edwin sometimes practices. Edwin maintained his assertion that flash cards might be too simplistic for his level of course work but agreed to try out both skills to study for an upcoming test—agreeing that the act of creating study tools might better engage him in the process.

In-Session Exercise: Introduce This Week's Skill Experiment ✪

Refer to "Structure of the Universal Skill Module" for instructions on how to introduce a weekly skill experiment. Using Worksheet 6.16, the family and the therapist can discuss adaptation of active studying skills for an upcoming test. The therapist can lead the teen and parent in a discussion to determine what test will be studied for, what days studying will occur, how long studying will occur daily, and which specific study activities are planned on each day.

Therapeutic Progress

Edwin decided to create a study plan for an upcoming advanced placement chemistry test. He indicated feeling confident about the math portion of the exam but expressed a desire to prepare carefully for the factual material on the test. His test was the following Monday—in exactly 1 week. Edwin said that his test was on three chapters of material and that he would use his class notes and textbook to prepare for the test. He decided to make reading notes for one chapter a night on Tuesday, Wednesday, and Thursday. On Saturday, Edwin would devote the entire afternoon to converting reading and class notes into flash cards. Finally, Edwin indicated that he would go through his flash cards on Sunday until he felt that he had mastered them and would do so again on Monday morning before the test. At the end of this planning, Edwin repeated his concern that he would not be able to overcome his motivation difficulties to enact the plan. The therapist asked him a scaling question to encourage Edwin to offer change talk in favor of successful studying, and in return Edwin cited the benefits of this plan as being less boring than his typical approach. The therapist also reminded Edwin of the time management skills discussed in the previous session—particularly how to break tasks into small steps to make it feel easier to get started.

While discussing the study plan, Maxine chimed in to ask Edwin where he planned to complete his studying. He said that he expected to study in his bedroom, and Maxine offered to talk to the other family members about keeping quiet and not disturbing Edwin while he was working. Edwin politely asked Maxine if she thought it would be fair for him to go over to his girlfriend's house for an hour before bed if he completed his daily studying before 9:00 P.M. She agreed, with the provision that if he didn't finish studying, he would need to stay home. Edwin offered to let Maxine hold the keys to his car until after he finished studying; Maxine replied that she trusted Edwin and believed that level of control was not necessary for a 17-year-old.

In a group setting, it may be appropriate to cover more than one skill module in a single session. All group sessions begin with a joint home activity review from the last session.

Parent Content: Using the subgroup discussion format, parents can discuss their ideas about successful ways to study and what methods their teens currently use to prepare for tests. The therapist can introduce the concept of active studying and can demonstrate for the parents how to use flash cards and take notes from text. The parents can try these skills for themselves as part of this procedure. Worksheets 6.12–6.15 can be employed to facilitate these discussions.

Teen Content: Teens can discuss their current challenges with studying and the strategies they use to prepare for tests and quizzes. Worksheets 6.12–6.15 can be used as the therapist introduces the concept of active studying and leads the teens to practice the flash cards and notes from text activities.

Collaborative Content ○: Teens and parents can work together to complete Worksheet 6.16 to detail a plan for studying for an upcoming test.

FIGURE 6.9. Delivering skill module 5 as a group.

Instead, they decided that Edwin would give his mother an update on his studying each night before 9:00 P.M.

Home Exercise: Implement Weekly Skill Experiment

The family should follow the contract detailed on Worksheet 6.16 for 1 week.

Skill Module 6: Note Taking

Checklist for Skill Module 6

Materials

☐ None

Worksheets

☐ Worksheet 6.17. Note-Taking Practice Sheet
☐ Worksheet 6.18. Note-Taking Contract

Case Example for Skill Module 6: Felicia and Anthony

Anthony is a 15-year-old in eighth grade at a local public middle school. He has an IEP that places him in a regular education setting with pullout services for math and reading. Anthony was held back in kindergarten and failed sixth grade, largely due to disruptive behavior and failure to complete work. His mother, Felicia, reports no involvement in academics, stating that Anthony is old enough to make his own decisions. Anthony and Felicia chose the note-taking module in hopes of improving Anthony's classroom behavior and academic engagement.

Review of Weekly Skill Experiment

Refer to "Structure of the Universal Skill Module" for instructions on how to conduct a review of the weekly skill experiment.

Progress Review

Refer to "Structure of the Universal Skill Module" for instructions on how to conduct a progress review.

Discussion: Introduce Skill

Refer to "Structure of the Universal Skill Module" for instructions on how to conduct skill introduction. The central topic of this EPE-style discussion is how EF or attention deficits can lead to difficulties staying on task in class and how off-task

KEY POINT: Off-Task Classroom Behavior

Teens with attention, EF, or motivation problems may experience difficulties in their ability to attend to and encode information and then store it until it is needed. In addition, when the teen finds a class to be boring or difficult, he or she may experience motivation problems during class. These motivation difficulties may make the teen attend to distractions rather than to class material. When attertnion and encoding skills are impaired, teens may have trouble focusing on classroom activities and remembering information that was presented in class without compensatory skills.

KEY POINT: Benefits of Note Taking

Note taking in class is a particularly beneficial skill for adolescents with attention or EF problems. Though some teachers may not require or even encourage note taking in their classes, performing this skill anyway may be highly beneficial to teens. These benefits are several.

Retention. The primary benefit of note taking is that it promotes attending to and storing information presented in class.

Distractibility. When adolescents take notes, they are more likely to remain on task during lectures, reducing interference by distractions.

Classroom behavior. When adolescents take notes in class, they are less likely to display disruptive behaviors in the classroom.

Test preparation. Taking notes in class provides the adolescent with a useful study guide for upcoming tests and quizzes.

Relationship with the teacher. When a teacher sees an adolescent taking notes in class, he or she may develop the impression that the adolescent is studious and takes academic work seriously.

behavior influences storage and retention of material. The key skill is taking notes in class.

Therapeutic Progress

Anthony was initially opposed to the idea of spending a session working on the skill of note taking, stating that it would be a waste of time. Felicia indicated that she felt strongly that note taking in class could be a realistic solution to Anthony's history of clowning around in class, refusing to comply with teacher requests, and opting out of classwork. She revealed a strong worry that he would fail the year, likening his current performance to his first sixth-grade year, when he was retained. The therapist affirmed Anthony's willingness to continue showing up to his classes, despite disliking his teachers. Anthony said that he continues to go to class because he does not want to fail the year but was starting to get aggravated with his teachers for criticizing him in front of his peers. In light of this information, the therapist reframed the session's purpose to finding ways to keep the teachers from singling him out during class. Anthony indicated that he could not think of any ways to improve his relationship with his teachers and that he felt ashamed of being the oldest student in his class. The therapist suggested that perhaps note taking would be a way to keep the teachers from criticizing him. Anthony remained unconvinced but agreed to participate in the session.

In-Session Exercise: Create Practice Plan

Refer to "Structure of the Universal Skill Module" for instructions on how to create a practice plan with the family. Adolescents may have varying degrees of note-taking skills, meaning that some adolescents need note-taking practice before they are able to apply this skill successfully in the classroom. Other teens may be skilled at note taking but may choose not to use this skill in their classes. To help the family assess whether note-taking skill development is needed, the therapist can conduct a note-taking assessment. This note-taking assessment doubles as a discussion of how note taking works. While the therapist presents material on how note taking works, the teen should be instructed to take notes on Worksheet 6.17.

The therapist can pause after each section of the notes (see Figure 6.10 on the next page) and offer feedback to the teen on his or her note-taking performance (with permission from the teen).

Therapeutic Progress

The therapist guided Anthony through the note-taking activity, offering feedback as he took notes on the material. Though Anthony's handwriting was difficult to understand, the content of his notes was adequate, indicating that he possessed the skills necessary to complete basic class notes. The therapist affirmed Anthony's abilities and intelligence and asked him whether he would be open to taking notes at least once during the upcoming week. With permission, the therapist suggested that Anthony do this in his least favorite class to see how his teacher would react. Anthony agreed to try it once but stated that he doubted his teacher would notice.

In-Session Exercise: Introduce This Week's Skill Experiment ✪

Refer to "Structure of the Universal Skill Module" for instructions on how to introduce a weekly skill experiment. Worksheet 6.18 is a contract template for skill module 6.

Therapeutic Progress

Anthony agreed that he would take notes in civics class once during the upcoming week. He noted that his civics teacher frequently scolds him in class. His mother

When delivering the lecture below to the teen, the therapist should attempt to imitate the pace and style of a typical secondary school teacher. To do so, the therapist should refrain from reading notes verbatim but, rather, should keep the lecture conversational and make the key points in his or her own words.

  I. When to take notes
     A. When teacher is presenting new material
     B. When teacher is reviewing for a test
     C. When you feel tempted to misbehave in class

 II. Benefits of note taking
     A. Soak in more material
     B. Obtain better grades on tests
     C. Become less distracted in class
     D. Less misbehavior
     E. Teacher will be impressed

III. What to listen for
     A. Main ideas—the central topics presented by the teacher
     B. Supporting details—information that describes main ideas
     C. Key words from teacher
        i. This is important
        ii. This word will be on the test

IV. Good note-taking habits
     A. Organize material on page with supporting details listed under main ideas
     B. Find ways to shorten words and sentences
     C. Leave out words that are not necessary
     D. Draw diagrams and pictures
     E. Only include the most important information

FIGURE 6.10. Note-taking lecture.

KEY POINT: Choosing a Class for Note Taking

For the weekly skill experiment, the family should choose one class in which the adolescent will take notes. One class (vs. multiple) is recommended to allow the teen to slowly introduce the skill into his or her daily routine. In choosing which class to designate for note taking, the family should consider why they selected the module (e.g., to improve retention, reduce distractibility, improve classroom behavior, enhance test preparation, improve the student's relationship with the teacher). The family should also consider whether the structure of the class lends itself to note taking.

In a group setting, it may be appropriate to cover more than one skill module in a single session. All group sessions begin with a joint home activity review from the last session.

Parent Content: Using the subgroup discussion format, parents can discuss common difficulties experienced by teens in the classroom. The therapist can ask the parents to discuss the skill of note taking, including their own experiences using this skill when they were students. Parents can brainstorm ideas for creating accountability at home for note taking at school.

Teen Content: Teens can discuss the benefits of note taking and past experiences using this skill. The therapist can deliver a lecture and ask the adolescents to take notes. The therapist can partner adolescents and ask them to provide peer feedback on notes. The therapist can make a list on the board of note-taking tips generated by the teens.

Collaborative Content ✪: Teens and parents can work together to complete Worksheet 6.18 to detail a plan for note taking in one class during the upcoming week.

FIGURE 6.11. Delivering skill module 6 in a group.

supported his decision, noting that he currently has an F in civics. Anthony voiced a desire to take his notes on a sheet of paper that he would borrow from a classmate, since he currently does not carry supplies to class. His mother offered to buy him a notebook, but Anthony declined her suggestion. When Anthony explained that he would keep his notes in his pocket, his mother objected, and Anthony acquiesced to using a notebook. Felicia stated that she wanted the notes to be at least a page long and to be legible. The pair decided that on the day that Anthony took notes, he would show them to his mother before dinner, and she would allow him to use his cell phone in the evening—a device she removed from his possession a week ago.

Home Exercise: Implement Weekly Skill Experiment

The family should follow the contract detailed on Worksheet 6.18 for 1 week.

Skill Module 7: Problem Solving

Checklist for Skill Module 7

Materials

☐ None

Worksheets

☐ Worksheet 6.19. Problem Solving
☐ Worksheet 6.20. Home Contract Template

Case Example for Skill Module 7: Juliette and Justin

Justin is a 10th-grade male who lives with his mother and stepfather and attends regular classes at a public high school. Justin's parents complain that he spends too much time on homework because he works very slowly. His mother, Juliette, joins him in treatment. She does not report any homework helping behavior but indicates that she frequently checks on Justin during homework time and finds him off task. Juliette reports frequent arguments with Justin when she attempts to redirect him back to his homework. Justin complains that he is easily distracted in his house because noises from his pets, parents, and the television prevent him from focusing on his work. In response to these concerns, Justin and Juliette completed a homework contract but reported that the enjoyable activity Justin was to earn (video games after homework) was not practical because Justin often does homework right until bedtime. The family decided to conduct a problem-solving module to give greater attention to this challenge.

Review of Weekly Skill Experiment

Refer to "Structure of the Universal Skill Module" for instructions on how to conduct a review of the weekly skill experiment.

Progress Review

Refer to "Structure of the Universal Skill Module" for instructions on how to conduct a progress review.

Discussion: Introduce Skill

Refer to "Structure of the Universal Skill Module" for instructions on how to conduct skill introduction. The central topic of this EPE-style discussion can be how EF or attention deficits can lead to difficulties making decisions when faced with a challenge. The key skill is using a problem-solving strategy to carefully think through decisions and plan how to act. See Figure 6.12.

KEY POINT: Planning and Decision Making

Teens with attention, EF, or motivation problems may experience difficulties coordinating goal-directed behavior. Specifically, they may experience difficulty using memory to store and compare multiple response options, as well as evaluating which response is most likely to lead to the desired outcome. These processes influence one's ability to understand a problematic situation, form a goal, and execute the goal with a well-formed plan. When these skills are impaired in teens, they may have trouble with decision making without compensatory skills.

DEFINE the problem. In this step, the teen writes a description of what is happening and what he or she hopes to accomplish by solving the problem. The teen can also write down why he or she thinks the problem is happening.

BRAINSTORM ideas. In this step the teen should list any ideas he or she has for ways to solve the problem. The therapist should encourage the teen to brainstorm as many ideas as possible, even if he or she is not sure if the ideas will work. Once the ideas are listed, the teen can write down the pros and cons of each one.

SOLUTION. In the final step, the teen can review the pros and cons listed and decide how he or she thinks the problem should be handled. This ultimate solution may include a combination of the ideas evaluated in the previous step.

FIGURE 6.12. Problem-solving steps.

In-Session Exercise: Create Practice Plan

Refer to "Structure of the Universal Skill Module" for instructions on how to create a practice plan with the family. To demonstrate this approach, the therapist can conduct a sample written problem evaluation with the family. Referring to Worksheet 6.19, the therapist can walk the teen through each step of the process.

During the sample problem-solving exercise, the family can be prompted to choose an issue with which they are currently struggling but that has not yet been addressed in treatment. This problem should be something the family thinks they can take steps to solve during the next week. For example, in Figure 6.13 Justin defines the issue.

Once the issue is defined, Justin and Juliette proceed by brainstorming several possible solutions and clearly articulating their pros and cons (see Figure 6.14 on the next page).

In the end, Justin and Juliette decide to combine aspects of several of the solutions above to arrive upon a possible way of addressing their predicament (see Figure 6.15).

In-Session Exercise: Introduce This Week's Skill Experiment

Refer to "Structure of the Universal Skill Module" for instructions on how to introduce a weekly skill experiment. Worksheet 6.20 is a contract template for skill module 7.

DEFINE

What is the issue?

I don't have enough time to enjoy my video game time in the evening because by the time I finish my homework, it's really late and it's time for bed. So I don't see the point in the contracts. I want to be able to actually get to play video games.

FIGURE 6.13. Defining the issue.

Ideas?	Pros	Cons
Stop homework early.	I will always have some time to relax.	I might not get homework done.
Start homework earlier in the car.	I might get some work done before I get home.	The car is distracting because of my sister.
Mom talks to school about how much homework I get.	They might give me less work so it won't take me so long to do it.	I don't know if they are allowed to give me less work.
I get to save up my video game time for weekend.	At least I still get it.	I don't really want to wait that long.
I can start homework earlier by going to the library right after school.	I can get started earlier and it's quiet there.	I might not be finished when the library closes.
I can do my video game time in the morning.	I will get my video game time.	It might make me late to school.

FIGURE 6.14. Considering alternatives.

SOLUTION

We decided to try out the library option for a week. It might be a way for me to focus better and get started earlier on homework. When the library closes at 8:00 P.M. mom will pick me up. She will see if I've finished my homework. If I have, then I can go play video games when we get home. If I haven't, I'll have to finish my homework at home and save the video games for the weekend. We are also going to schedule a meeting with the counselor to talk about why the work is taking me so long to get done.

FIGURE 6.15. Arriving upon a solution.

In a group setting, it may be appropriate to cover more than one skill module in a single session. All group sessions begin with a joint home activity review from the last session.

Parent Content: Parents can learn the problem-solving steps and work through a sample problem together in a large- or small-group format.

Teen Content: Teens can also learn the problem-solving steps, practicing these steps several times in their groups—at least once in a large-group setting and once in a small-group setting—until they can perform the steps independently.

Collaborative Content ✪: Teens and parents can work together to identify a problem and to complete Worksheet 6.19 to use the problem-solving steps to solve the problem. Finally, families can use the contract form on Worksheet 6.20 to devise a plan for implementing the solution.

FIGURE 6.16. Delivering skill module 7 in a group.

Therapeutic Progress

After completing the problem example displayed above, Justin indicated that he felt hopeful about doing his homework in the library because it would allow him to start his work earlier and stay in the school mind-set until his homework is completed. His mother expressed a concern that without her assistance, he might not organize himself to get started on work in the library; however, she agreed to restrict her role to picking him up from the library at 8:00 and checking his progress on homework at that time. Despite being unsure of whether the plan would improve Justin's homework performance, both agreed to observe and notice what happened when they tried the new approach.

Home Exercise: Implement Weekly Skill Experiment

The family should follow the contract detailed on Worksheet 6.20 for 1 week. In addition, the therapist can discuss with the family how they can use the problem-solving method to solve future problems that may arise at home. This approach can be combined with the family meeting skills (see engagement module 3) to create a parent–teen collaborative approach to managing problems.

1. Where might you write down or type in your homework assignments each day?

2. When might you decide to write down each assignment so you can make sure you don't forget?

3. What can you do if there is no homework to prove that you didn't just forget to write it down?

4. When should your parent check to see if you wrote down the assignments?

5. Should teachers get involved in this plan to check whether you have correctly recorded your homework?

(A) I will write down homework in the following location: _____.

For each class writing down homework will occur (circle one):

At the beginning of class   At the end of class   As soon as it's announced

If there is no homework, I will write: _____

The role I want my teachers to have in this is: _____

(B) Teen's list of enjoyable activities that must wait until after responsibility:

(C) Parent's role in reinforcing part (B):

(D) To promote independence, what parent will *not* do:

_____   _____
Teen Signature   Parent Signature

	Did teen do (A)?					Did parent do (C & D)?				
Day:	1	2	3	4	5	1	2	3	4	5
Y/N?										

1. How long does the student typically spend on homework each night? How long do you believe the student should be spending on homework each night?

2. What distractions must be removed from the homework environment to improve homework time?

3. What other challenges does the teen experience during homework time?

4. What is the parent's current role in homework time? What is the parent's desired role in homework time?

(A) I agree that homework time will occur (circle days that apply):

Monday   Tuesday   Wednesday   Thursday   Friday   Saturday   Sunday

I will start homework when: _____ and I will be allowed to stop

homework when: _____

The location of homework will be: _____

In order to create a distraction-free environment, we will: _____

_____

_____

Homework rules will be: _____

_____

_____

(B) Teen's list of enjoyable activities that must wait until after homework:

(C) Parent's role in reinforcing part (B):

(D) To promote independence, what parent will *not* do:

	Did teen do (A)?					Did parent do (C & D)?				
Day:	1	2	3	4	5	1	2	3	4	5
Y/N?										

There are several steps to finding organization and keeping it. All of these steps must occur in order for things to get organized and stay organized.

STEP 1: Clean out the mess!

- Throw away old papers, candy wrappers, and unnecessary trash.
- Put away clothes and things that have a proper place at home.
- Sort papers you want to keep by subject.

STEP 2: Decide upon an organization system.

- Do you want to use one big binder with lots of sections/folders in it?
- Do you want to create one binder for each block shedule day (if applicable)?
- Do you want to use one separate binder for each class?
- Should you use a homework folder to help locate homework quickly?
- Where should writing utensils be stored?

STEP 3: Create an organization checklist.

- Decide on what must be done to maintain organization.
- Write down a list with columns for each date (see sample in Worksheet 6.6).

STEP 4: Monitor organization.

- Decide how often organization will be monitored (daily, twice a week, etc.).
- Decide who will monitor organization.
- Agree upon criteria for decreasing frequency of monitoring (e.g., decreasing monitoring once a week as soon as teen gets 100% for 4 weeks straight).

WORKSHEET 6.6. Sample Organization Checkup Practice Plan

	Record Date Below					
Checkup Criteria						
1. All papers are in a secure folder or binder.						
2. There is a folder for each class with only papers for that class inside.						
3. There is a homework folder that contains all work that needs to be turned in.						
4. There are no clothes in the book bag.						
5. All pens and pencils are in the pencil case.						
Total Criteria Met:						

Check off all criteria that were met.

Checkup Criteria	Record Date Below					
1.						
2.						
3.						
4.						
5.						
Total Criteria Met:						

What new materials must be obtained in order to follow this plan?

What is our plan for obtaining them?

(A) I will monitor my book bag for organization on the following days next week (circle days when check will occur):

Monday   Tuesday   Wednesday   Thursday   Friday   Saturday   Sunday

The point in the day at which this checkup will occur is: _____

The number of items on my checklist that I must meet is: _____

If I miss an item on the checklist, the plan for correcting it will be: _____

_____

_____

(B) Teen's list of enjoyable activities that must wait until after responsibility:

(If checkups are not daily, consider using a point system to earn a long-term enjoyable activity.)

(C) Parent's role in reinforcing part (B):

(D) To promote independence, what parent will *not* do:

_____   _____
Teen Signature   Parent Signature

	Did teen do (A)?					Did parent do (C & D)?				
Day:	1	2	3	4	5	1	2	3	4	5
Y/N?										

Instructions: Break down the first step into smaller and smaller pieces until the first step feels easy to get started on. Sometimes people find that once they get started it is not as hard to keep going.

Example task: Write an essay

Small step: Write the first paragraph.

Smaller step: Write the first sentence of the first paragraph.

Now you try it: Think of a homework assignment you are not looking forward to. Break it down in the space below until you feel that the first step is easy enough that you feel ready to get started.

Task:

Small step:

Smaller step:

Even smaller step:

Tip: Use breaks to reward yourself for finishing a certain number of steps.

Date: _____

Order	Homework task	How long will it take?	Adult initials
	Tests/quizzes to study for		
	Long-term projects to work on		
	Online learning to complete		
	Reading to do		

Prioritizing

1. What tasks are due soonest? _____

2. What tasks are easiest to get started on? _____

3. What tasks are worth a lot of my grade? _____

(A) I will use time management strategies on the following days next week (circle days when check will occur):

Monday   Tuesday   Wednesday   Thursday   Friday   Saturday   Sunday

My time management strategy is to: _____

_____

_____

The point at which I show my list to my parent will be: _____

The point at which I will show my parent I've completed each assignment will be (circle one):

        after each assignment   after all assignments are done

(B) Teen's list of enjoyable activities that must wait until after responsibility:

(C) Parent's role in reinforcing part (B):

(D) To promote independence, what parent will *not* do:

_____   _____
Teen Signature   Parent Signature

	Did teen do (A)?					Did parent do (C & D)?				
Day:	1	2	3	4	5	1	2	3	4	5
Y/N?										

How do you typically study for tests and quizzes? _____

_____

_____

_____

_____

_____

_____

_____

_____

_____

_____

_____

_____

_____

_____

_____

_____

_____

_____

Research suggests that people learn better if they use active studying instead of passive studying.

Active Studying	Passive Studying
• *Doing* something with the information • Forcing your brain to store the information • Writing down information • Organizing information • Making and studying flash cards • Taking notes from textbook	• Looking at the information • Making it easy to daydream or stop paying attention • Staring at a textbook or set of notes • Reading over information • Having someone else quiz you

Especially Helpful for:

- Vocabulary tests
- Foreign language
- Remembering facts

How to Create Flash Cards:

- Put the word, person, event, or concept on one side.
- Put the definition, synonym, translation, or facts on the other side.
- **Limit the number of words on each side to four.**
  - Limiting the number of words forces you to mentally manipulate the material and find the perfect four words. This is the key to active studying!.

How to Study Flash Cards:

- Look at one side of the card and say out loud what you think is on the other side (without looking).
- If you are correct, put the card in pile 1.
- If you are incorrect, put the card in pile 2.
- Repeat this process until all of the cards in pile 2 have made it to pile 1.

How to Be Ready for the Test:

- Be able to go through your stack of flash cards in *3 seconds or less* per card. For example, you should be able to go through a stack of 20 cards in 1 minute.
- Take your cards to school the day of the test. Find time to review them for 5 minutes right before the test, in the morning before school starts, or at lunch.

Make a set of flash cards for the five pseudo-words below. Make sure to limit the number of words on each side of the flash card to four. See if you can go through your flash cards in under 15 seconds!

1. Borken—a rounded object used to mash potatoes

2. Batto—a child who is very attached to his mother

3. Hastize—to yell obscenities at someone who has made a horrible mistake

4. Throke—to eat a meal very quickly

5. Husp—warm clothing worn by a dog in the wintertime

Benefits of Notes from Text:

- Forces you to mentally manipulate material
- Creates a study guide that can be useful
- Writing down information helps your brain store it
- Prevents you from daydreaming while you are reading

How to Take Notes from Text:

- Read the paragraph.
- Find the main point of the paragraph and write it on the page.
- Underneath the main point, put the supporting details.
- Only write down important information.
- Use abbreviations.

Notes from Text Exercise:

Richard Nixon's childhood shaped who he became as president. He was raised in California during the 1920s. His parents were very poor. One of the sad things that happened during Nixon's childhood was that his brother died at the age of seven after a short illness. As president, Nixon never forgot these experiences.

Main Topic:

I. _____

Supporting Details:

A. _____

B. _____

C. _____

(A) The test I will study for is: _____ Test date: _____

Over the next week, I will complete the following study activities:

Day of the week: _____ What I will do: _____

_____

Day of the week: _____ What I will do: _____

_____

Day of the week: _____ What I will do: _____

_____

Day of the week: _____ What I will do: _____

_____

Day of the week: _____ What I will do: _____

_____

(B) Teen's list of enjoyable activities that must wait until after responsibility:

(C) Parent's role in reinforcing part (B):

(D) To promote independence, what parent will *not* do:

_____   _____
Teen Signature   Parent Signature

	Did teen do (A)?					Did parent do (C & D)?				
Day:	1	2	3	4	5	1	2	3	4	5
Y/N?										

_____

_____

_____

_____

_____

_____

_____

_____

_____

_____

_____

_____

_____

_____

_____

_____

(A) For the next week I will take notes in the following class: _____

These notes will be taken in a (circle one):   binder   sheet of paper   notebook that
will be kept: _____ .

My notes will be considered acceptable if they meet the following criteria:

(1)

(2)

(3)

(B) Teen's list of enjoyable activities that must wait until after responsibility:

(C) Parent's role in reinforcing part (B):

(D) To promote independence, what parent will *not* do:

_____   _____
Teen Signature   Parent Signature

	Did teen do (A)?					Did parent do (C & D)?				
Day:	1	2	3	4	5	1	2	3	4	5
Y/N?										

DEFINE

What is the issue?

_____

_____

_____

_____

_____

BRAINSTORM

Ideas?	Pros	Cons

SOLUTION

_____

_____

_____

_____

_____

_____

(A) Teen's daily responsibility:

(B) Teen's list of enjoyable activities that must wait until after responsibility:

(C) Parent's role in reinforcing part (B):

(D) To promote independence, what parent will *not* do:

_____   _____
Teen Signature   Parent Signature

	Did teen do (A)?					Did parent do (C & D)?				
Day:	1	2	3	4	5	1	2	3	4	5
Y/N?										

CHAPTER 7

Mobilizing Modules

Mobilizing modules are designed to consolidate what is learned in skill modules to create plans for moving forward. Skill modules expose teens to daily strategies to compensate for attention, EF, and motivation deficits. Mobilizing modules allow families to form long-term plans to integrate these skills into their daily lives.

During mobilizing sessions (see Figure 7.1), parents and teens discuss how to engage school staff in support of the teen's skill application at school. Families participate in a second focusing process of choosing skills to practice long term, integrating these skills into a home routine, and structuring the home environment to

---

Mobilizing Module 1: Engaging the School: The goal of this session is to discuss how to engage the teen's school in support of the teen's new habits. As part of this discussion, the parent and teen discuss their desired roles for school staff in supporting new skills, as well as strategies for building strong relationships with key school staff members.

Mobilizing Module 2: Habit Formation: The goal of this session is to plan a daily routine with the teen and parent that includes any new skills practiced during modular sessions, as well as completion of major daily responsibilities.

Mobilizing Module 3: Making an Action Plan: The purpose of this session is to select up to three skills or responsibilities that are not yet habits and create a parent–teen contract that serves as an action plan for the family moving forward.

Mobilizing Module 4: Keeping Momentum: The purpose of this session is to reflect upon changes made during treatment and to discuss strategies for maintaining changes long term.

FIGURE 7.1. Overview of mobilizing modules.

promote long-term practice. Mobilizing modules encourage families to reflect upon changes made during treatment and to identify strategies that maintain progress after treatment concludes.

Mobilizing Module 1: Engaging the School

Checklist for Mobilizing Module 1

Materials

- ☐ None

Worksheets

- ☐ Worksheet 7.1. How Can My School Help?
- ☐ Worksheet 7.2. Menu of Strategies to Engage School Staff
- ☐ Worksheet 7.3. School Conversation
- ☐ Worksheet 7.4. Next Steps

Topics

- ☐ Review of weekly skill experiment
- ☐ Progress review
- ☐ Desired school collaboration
- ☐ Identifying a point person
- ☐ Strategies for school staff engagement
- ☐ Outline conversation with school
- ☐ Consider next steps
- ☐ Introduce home exercise: Next Steps

Key MI Skills

- ☐ Use EPE to introduce activities and information about school collaboration.
- ☐ Elicit the benefits of engaging with the school.
- ☐ Emphasize the family's autonomy in choosing how to engage with the school.
- ☐ Query reasons for family choices about school collaboration. Promote elaboration.
- ☐ Listen for and reflect mobilizing change talk.

Case Example for Mobilizing Module 1: Roger and Madison

Madison is a seventh-grade student at a private middle school who comes to treatment with her father, Roger. Madison and Roger completed skill modules on writing down homework, creating a homework plan, and organization checkups. As part of these sessions, they decided to continue use of a daily planner, twice-weekly book bag organization checkups, and a structured homework routine. During skill modules, Roger struggled to consistently monitor Madison's planner use and rarely conducted scheduled book bag inspections. Roger and Madison decided that watching cartoons in the morning before school, which Madison commonly enjoys, would be allowed only after Madison has shown proof of all assignments written in her planner and fully completed homework. Roger reported inconsistent implementation of this plan, citing a hectic home schedule and forgetfulness as obstacles to consistent home structure.

Review of Weekly Skill Experiment

This component of the session is discussed in Chapter 6.

Progress Review

This component of the session is discussed in Chapter 6.

Discussion: Desired School Collaboration

The therapist can begin the session by asking the family to share their viewpoints on family–school partnership. Following this discussion, the therapist can ask permission to explore ways in which coordination with the school might promote monitoring and reinforcement of independent skill practice.

To guide this discussion, the parent and teen can refer to Worksheet 7.1, which asks family members to recall the skills that they are practicing, which aspects of skills occur in the school setting, how feedback on skill use in the school setting might be helpful to the parent and teen, and how collaboration with the school might be useful in promoting teen skill use.

During this conversation, the therapist can emphasize parent and teen autonomy in deciding what level and type of school involvement would be best for the family. At the same time, the therapist can listen for and reinforce change talk related to goals set by the family in engagement module 2. Though some families may be hesitant to collaborate with the school, some level of school coordination is likely to enhance monitoring of teen progress.

Therapeutic Progress

During the discussion of school collaboration, Roger indicated that he finds Madison's school very helpful and expressed a preference to have the therapist work directly with the school—removing his own involvement. He explained that the school typically initiates communication with him and his wife as needed and that he did not remember a time that he proactively made contact with the school. Throughout the discussion, Roger nudges Madison to respond to the therapist's

KEY POINTS: Developmental Considerations

The secondary school academic environment differs drastically from that of elementary school in that students are expected to function more independently and navigate multiple classes each day. Secondary school teachers often teach 100 or more students, leaving them with less available time per student than elementary school teachers. Similarly, middle and high school counselors often carry a caseload of 500 to 1,000 students. Effective engagement of secondary school staff must consider the realities of these environmental constraints. Based on our work coordinating home–school collaboration with families, key considerations are listed below.

Formalize supports. Eligible families should consider obtaining documented accommodations through their school system (e.g., individualized education plan, Section 504 plan), which may increase the likelihood that school staff will devote extra time and resources to student support.

Engage nonteaching staff. Engaging a special educator may be more successful than engaging a school counselor, which in turn is likely to be more successful than engaging a classroom teacher. Special educators are often assigned to intervention provision as a part of their job responsibilities. School counselors are free from the constraints of teaching consecutive classes and may have more flexibility to meet with students or coordinate with multiple teachers.

Brief interventions. Support activities that take very little staff time are typically more likely to be implemented than intensive interventions. These services require fewer school resources and can be delivered without removing the student from the classroom setting.

Appropriate communication. Regular parent–school communication enhances progress monitoring and school willingness to help; however, overly frequent communication (i.e., more than one contact per week with a staff member) may be viewed as burdensome and may damage rapport with secondary school staff. Parents and teens should discuss appropriate levels of parent–school communication with the school staff prior to intervention coordination.

Promote independence. Expectations for adolescent independence are an embedded component of the secondary school culture. Staff may be most likely to accept interventions when their stated purpose is to require independent work completion from the teen. Staff also may be more likely to participate in monitoring or skill reinforcement when the teen plays an active role in these processes.

Honor staff expertise. Just as the parent and teen are experts on their family, school staff are experts on their school. Thus parent and teen deference to this expertise is a key component of successful school staff engagement.

Involve the teen. Teen involvement in discussions with teachers, IEP and 504 plan meetings, and school intervention formulation is appropriate at the secondary school level. Parents and teens should be encouraged to engage equally in this process and to advocate for adolescent involvement when teachers prefer the adolescent to be absent.

questions—even those directed at him as a parent. He also blames Madison for a lack of progress in therapy. Noticing Roger's continued belief that change should come from the teen rather than the parent, the therapist makes marked attempts to elicit from Roger desire and reasons to increase his parental involvement. In the end, Roger concedes that monitoring whether Madison writes in her planner would be a reasonable role for him as a parent and hesitantly offers that coordinating with teachers about Madison's planner use might be useful. Due to Roger's continued ambivalence about his involvement in providing structure at home, the therapist will continue to elicit and strengthen change talk from Roger about his influence on Madison's behavior.

Discussion: *Identifying a Point Person*

As a part of the school engagement process, it is beneficial for families to collaborate with a school employee who can serve as liaison between home and school. Given the complexity of secondary school environments, engaging a point person allows the family to build rapport with a specific individual who may be able to monitor and communicate about student skill use and progress at school. Using EPE (see Chapter 4), the therapist can describe the idea of a point person and discuss with the parent and teen the benefits of engaging a school staff member as a special contact at the school. The therapist and the family can brainstorm potential school staff members to serve as the point person.

Once the family has identified a candidate, the therapist can use open-ended questions and reflections to elicit change talk about the benefits of working with the identified staff member, as well as the promise of building rapport with a specific point person at the school.

Therapeutic Progress

The therapist introduced the notion of a point person, and Roger explained that Madison has an academic advisor who is expected to serve as a point of contact for the parent. Madison revealed that she feels unacquainted with her advisor, who does not teach her in a class and only meets with her advisory group once a month.

> **KEY POINT:** *Choosing a Point Person*
>
> When considering who can serve as an effective point person, the family should identify individuals with whom the student has rapport and who may be available and willing to serve as a liaison for the family. It is important to consider whether the staff member's job responsibilities align with the desired type of assistance. Special education staff members (when the student has an IEP) are typically the most successful point people, followed by school counselors and then classroom teachers. However, there may be alternatives in unique situations, such as a coach, an aide, or an administrator with whom the student has a special relationship.

When asked to name someone who might be a more helpful point person, Madison suggested the support teacher at her school who offers special assistance to students with academic difficulties. After eliciting minor change talk from skeptical Roger about the potential benefits of collaborating with this support teacher, the pair agreed to contact the support teacher.

In-Session Exercise: Strategies for School Staff Engagement

Once a point person has been considered, the therapist can guide the parent and teen through a conversation about strategies for engaging school staff. The therapist can refer to Worksheet 7.2, which lists a menu of strategies to engage school staff, as well as Figure 7.2.

Therapeutic Progress

Reviewing the menu of strategies (see Worksheet 7.2), Roger informed the therapist that he occasionally e-mails Madison's teachers when he has a question about her academic progress. He noted that he feels compelled to e-mail a teacher if he finds out that Madison has a poor grade in a class and explained that he likes to address poor grades as soon as he finds out about them. The therapist affirmed this intention. Madison added that she enjoyed giving gifts to her favorite teachers, and Roger agreed with the importance of showing gratitude when a teacher has gone out of her way to assist Madison. Roger also expressed appreciation for another menu item— recognizing teacher concerns—stating that he felt it was important for parents not to deny that their child is having academic difficulties. Near the end of this discussion, the therapist asked Madison which strategies she might find helpful in asking her teachers for support with her daily planner. Madison replied that it would be helpful for her teachers to check whether she had correctly written down her homework assignments, but that she might need to politely ask them to do so each day, as teachers are often busy at the end of class.

Step 1: Emphasize the family's autonomy by stating that there is no best practice for engaging school staff. Encourage family to formulate their own unique strategy.

Step 2: Introduce the menu as a list of strategies that have helped other families in the past.

Step 3: Ask the parent and teen to review the menu and identify strategies they found helpful in the past.

Step 4: Elicit change talk about the benefits of any identified engagement approach. Help the parent and teen look ahead to how the engagement approach might benefit their current situation.

Step 5: Ask the family to consider new strategies on the menu that could be potentially useful.

Step 6: Elicit change talk about the benefits of the new approaches.

FIGURE 7.2. Steps for reviewing the school engagement strategy menu.

In-Session Exercise: Outline Conversation with School ✪

Referring to Worksheet 7.3, the therapist can ask the family to brainstorm a hypothetical conversation with the school. With the family's permission, the therapist can guide the family through this worksheet, discussing points the parent would like to make during the meeting, points the adolescent would like to make during the meeting, affirmations that the family would like to give to the school staff members, questions the parent and teen would like to ask the school staff members, and strategies that the parent and teen think would be helpful during the meeting with school staff. After the details are gathered, the therapist can ask the parent and teen to reflect upon what they think would happen if they held such a meeting, reflecting change talk about the benefits of doing so.

Therapeutic Progress

The pair outlined the points they would like to make at a potential meeting with Madison's support teacher. Madison stated that she would like to improve her planner use and would ask her teacher to help coordinate a way for her to get teacher initials in her planner each day. With the therapist's assistance, Madison practiced a sentence she might say to the support teacher to explain her difficulties: "I'm trying hard in school but sometimes I forget what my homework is and I end up with missing work." Roger offers that the support teacher has a reputation for going above and beyond for students—and that he will thank her for this during the meeting. To clarify what is feasible, he also suggested that he ask the support teacher whether it is realistic for Madison to expect that her teachers will sign off on her planner each day.

Discussion: Consider Next Steps

At this point in the session, the therapist can ask the parent and the teen what they think they will do next to engage the school. Once again, the therapist can emphasize that only the family can know what would be the best thing to do in their particular situation. As part of this discussion, the therapist can identify mobilizing change talk related to specific actions that the family plans to take. The therapist can ask for elaboration on why these steps were chosen and exactly how they will be carried out. On Worksheet 7.4, the family can write down their next steps, including something concrete they each can do in the next week.

Therapeutic Progress

Roger makes a commitment to e-mail the support teacher to set up a meeting. He pulls out his phone in session to do so immediately. Madison agrees to stop by the

All group sessions begin with a joint home activity review from the last session.

Parent Content: Using the subgroup discussion format, parents can be prompted to discuss desired school involvement, past experiences working with the school, how to choose a point person, and strategies that successfully engage teachers. Worksheets 7.1 and 7.2 support these discussions.

Teen Content: Teens can also discuss the type of support they would like from school staff, as well as strategies for developing good relationships with teachers. The therapist can complete Worksheets 7.1 and 7.2 with teens.

Collaborative Content ☸: Parents and teens complete Worksheet 7.3, which asks them to devise a plan for a school meeting with a potential point person.

FIGURE 7.3. Delivering mobilizing module 1 in a group.

teacher's office the following morning to mention that her father sent an e-mail. To close the conversation, the therapist asks the pair what they hope will be the outcome of their actions. Roger states that he hopes that Madison will take the initiative to use her planner more often as a result of the school meeting. When prompted for a more personal response, Roger paused and acknowledged that having the meeting might be a good first step for him to start over with his attempts to set structure at home. Anticipating that Roger may not complete the home exercise due to his past inconsistency, the therapist plans to affirm any positive efforts made by Roger during the next session, continuing to elicit change talk about the benefits of creating structure at home for Madison.

Home Exercise: Next Steps

The therapist can direct the parent's and teen's attention to Worksheet 7.4. The parent and teen can be asked whether they are willing to try implementation of their next steps during the upcoming week. With the parent's and teen's permission, the therapist can affirm the family's choices for next steps.

Mobilizing Module 2: Habit Formation

Checklist for Mobilizing Module 2

Materials

☐ None

Worksheets

☐ Worksheet 7.5. Toolbox

☐ Worksheet 7.6. Building a Daily Routine

Topics

- ☐ Discuss efforts to engage school
- ☐ Progress review
- ☐ Skills versus habits
- ☐ Loading the toolbox
- ☐ Building a daily routine
- ☐ Introduce home exercise: Implement Habit-Tracking Plan

Key MI Skills

- ☐ Use EPE to introduce new information.
- ☐ Emphasize family member autonomy in choosing desired habits.
- ☐ Elicit change talk from the parent and teen about turning skills into habits.
- ☐ Provide affirmations about family member efforts toward habit formation.

Case Example for Mobilizing Module 2: Ingrid and Louisa

Louisa is a ninth-grade student who attends a small charter school and is placed in regular classes. She and her mother, Ingrid, completed skill modules on writing down homework, study skills, and problem solving. The problem-solving session was selected because Louisa struggles to complete her supplementary online math and reading homework. Over the course of treatment, Louisa showed progress in her consistent use of a daily planner and study skills, and Ingrid consistently checked Louisa's planner and monitored study time. Each day, after Louisa showed appropriate planner use and studying, she was allowed to use her cell phone. Ingrid appropriately asked for Louisa's cell phone as soon as she returned from school each day and held it until the next day if Louisa did not complete her tasks. During mobilizing module 1, Ingrid expressed a desire to talk to the ninth-grade counselor. She hoped to schedule a meeting with the counselor and all of Louisa's teachers to discuss her progress. Ingrid's principal hope was to open communication about whether Louisa was doing her online homework.

Discussion: Efforts to Engage School

The therapist can begin the session by discussing the parent's and teen's efforts during the previous week to engage school staff, as outlined by the family in mobilizing module 1. As part of this discussion, the therapist can affirm all family efforts, regardless of their magnitude or success. The therapist can also reflect change talk related to parent and teen hopes for school engagement or continued efforts to engage the school. Many families experience difficulties making contact with school staff. It may take many weeks to establish contact and set a meeting. The therapist should normalize concerns that the school was not immediately responsive.

Therapeutic Progress

During review of the home exercise, Ingrid said that she had left Louisa's counselor three phone messages but had not yet received a response. Louisa, who had previously committed to stopping by her counselor's office, stated that she could not find her during the past week. When prompted for next steps, Ingrid decided that she would go to the school in person to ask for the counselor. Louisa begged her mother not to visit the school, stating that it would embarrass her. The pair agreed that Louisa would be given a chance to find the counselor herself and would ask her to call her mother on the spot. By the end of the week, if Louisa's efforts were unsuccessful, Ingrid stated that she would visit the school. The therapist affirmed the family for using a problem-solving approach and respectful communication skills to compromise on an appropriate solution.

Progress Review

This component of the session is described in Chapter 6.

Discussion: Skills versus Habits

Using EPE (see Chapter 4), the therapist can ask the family to share their views on the difference between skills and habits. As part of this conversation, the therapist

---

KEY POINTS: How Do Habits Form?

The process of starting a new habit is outlined below.

1. Habits start with a decision to repeat a new skill. Deciding to form a habit requires having a good reason to do so.
2. Once the decision is made, daily practice is required to help the skill become automatic.
3. Once a skill becomes automatic, it takes less effort to remember and complete the skill. Therefore, the more the teen (or parent) practices the skill, the easier it will be to remember and complete it each day.

Habit formation can be especially difficult for teens with attention, EF, and motivation deficits. To promote habit formation, the therapist can consider the following:

1. MI conversations that elicit from the teen the benefits of skill use can strengthen the teen's desire to form a habit. Witnessing the benefits of weekly skill experiments with one's own eyes can further strengthen reasons to practice.
2. Structure that requires responsibilities to come before enjoyable activities can promote daily skill practice that leads to habit formation. Parent involvement is needed to maintain this structure.
3. Habit formation can take time. It may take weeks or months for teen skill use to become automatic. The family should not give up if skill practice is initially inconsistent.

can query activities that the parent and teen do every day that they consider habits. The parent and teen can be asked to reflect upon how they turned these responsibilities into habits.

Therapeutic Progress

Ingrid and Louisa discussed the automaticity of habits, and Louisa acknowledged that having good daily hygiene was the responsibility that she had most ingrained into habit. In this discussion, Louisa identified that caring about how she is perceived by peers is the reason she is motivated to have good hygiene. Ingrid recalled that when Louisa was in elementary school she would have to prompt her to take a shower or brush her teeth, but by middle school Louisa completed these responsibilities without reminders. The two agreed that having a good reason to practice something daily is a big factor in developing habits.

In-Session Exercise: Loading the Toolbox

Using Worksheet 7.5 as a guide, the therapist can ask the parent and the teen to consider the skills that they have each practiced since beginning treatment. The therapist can encourage the parent and the teen to write down all skills in their respective toolboxes on Worksheet 7.5 (see Figure 7.4). While eliciting these skills, the therapist can ask the parent and the teen to share their reasons for wanting to turn these skills into habits and what they expect will happen if they are successful at doing so. As a part of this exercise, the parent and teen should each circle skills they would like

---

Sample Teen Toolbox (Louisa)

Taking deep breaths when my mom upsets me
"I" statements
Putting responsibilities before fun activities
Writing down homework assignments in a planner
Flash cards
Reading notes

Sample Parent Toolbox (Ingrid)

"I" statements
Holding a parent–teen meeting
Checking her planner every day
Taking possession of her cell phone until she finishes her responsibilities
E-mailing the teachers (hopefully) to coordinate about online learning

---

FIGURE 7.4. Sample teen and parent toolboxes.

to turn into automatic habits. Reviewing engagement module 2 treatment goals is a helpful way to help families decide on which skills they would like to prioritize. The therapist can listen for preparatory and mobilizing change talk during this discussion and can reflect these statements to encourage elaboration and deepening of the desire to form new habits.

Therapeutic Progress

During the toolbox activity, Ingrid states that she would like to make an automatic habit of checking Louisa's planner each day and obtaining her cell phone after school. The therapist responds to these desires by linking them to Ingrid's wish to see Louisa become more organized and productive at home and school. Louisa agreed that she hopes to make a habit of writing in her planner, studying for tests, and completing her online learning each day. When prompted to explain her choices, Louisa stated that the most important reason to complete these tasks was to get her phone back from her mother. The therapist reaffirms Ingrid's efforts to create consistent structure at home that motivates Louisa to succeed: Just as Louisa was motivated by peer opinion to turn good hygiene into a habit, she appeared to be motivated by cell phone use to turn good organization into a habit. The family appreciated this comparison and seemed optimistic for continued progress in therapy.

In-Session Exercise: Building a Daily Routine ✪

Using Worksheet 7.6, the therapist can begin working with the family to plan out a daily routine that encourages daily skill practice. With the family's permission, the therapist can ask family members to organize desired daily habits from the Worksheet 7.5 toolbox by time of day (morning, school day, evening) on Worksheet 7.6. The therapist can also ask the parent and teen to add any additional responsibilities (e.g., household chores, academic tasks) that they would like to build into a daily routine. The therapist can use EPE to explain that over the next week, family

---

KEY POINTS: Taking Time Each Day to Notice Skill Use

The daily routine home exercise works best if tasks are noticed and recorded daily. This requires parents to take a moment from each day and to notice whether or not the parent and teen completed their tasks.

Some parents and teens wait until the end of the week to retrospectively report whether skill use occurred. As a preventative measure, the therapist may engage the parent and teen in a conversation about how to make sure that information on the worksheet is accurate— perhaps by planning a nightly parent–teen meeting about whether tasks occurred, posting the list in an easily viewable location, or setting a phone reminder to complete the list daily.

members can work together to track whether or not each task occurred each day. In the upcoming session, progress toward habit formation will be discussed.

No formal contract is enacted for the home exercise detailed on Worksheet 7.6. This is purposeful to allow the family to collect naturalistic data on the teen's (and parent's) progress toward naturalistic habit formation. This information is especially helpful in mobilizing module 3 when the family is building an action plan for moving forward.

Therapeutic Progress

When preparing for the daily routine home exercise, Louisa and Ingrid discuss whether they should continue to keep their new structure at home. The therapist offered that some families decide to remove structure for a week (in this case, having the cell phone wait until after responsibilities are complete) to determine which tasks were already habits. Ingrid voiced a desire to keep the cell phone structure in place so that she could continue to practice implementing it. The therapist and family agreed that in this case, it made sense to continue with the home structure they had been practicing for the last few weeks.

Home Exercise: Implement Habit-Tracking Plan

The therapist can direct the parent's and teen's attention to Worksheet 7.6. The parent and teen can be asked whether they are willing to keep track of skills they practice during the upcoming week. The parent and teen can indicate whether the tasks were completed, not completed, or unknown. One important aspect of this exercise is helping parents realize which tasks are possible to monitor. Tasks about which the parent does not have daily information may not be appropriate for inclusion in the upcoming action plan (see mobilizing module 3).

All group sessions begin with a joint home activity review from the last session.

Parent Content: Using the subgroup discussion format, parents can be prompted to discuss the meaning of skills versus habits, past experiences turning skills into habits, and which skills and responsibilities they would like to turn into habits. Worksheet 7.5 can be used to support these discussions.

Teen Content: Teens can also discuss the difference between skills and habits, as well as the skills and responsibilities they hope to turn into habits. The therapist can complete Worksheet 7.5 with teens.

Collaborative Content ✪: Parents and teens complete Worksheet 7.6, which asks them to identify habits for tracking in the next week.

FIGURE 7.5. Delivering mobilizing module 2 in a group.

Mobilizing Module 3: Making an Action Plan

Checklist for Mobilizing Module 3

Materials

- ☐ None

Worksheets

- ☐ Worksheet 7.7. Action Plan Ideas
- ☐ Worksheet 7.8. Action Plan
- ☐ Worksheet 7.9. Action Plan Log

Topics

- ☐ Discuss building a daily routine
- ☐ Progress review
- ☐ Forming an action plan
- ☐ How to structure an action plan
- ☐ Create an action plan
- ☐ Home exercise: Implement an action plan

Key MI Skills

- ☐ Use EPE to present information to family.
- ☐ Emphasize family choice in designing action plans.
- ☐ Listen for and reflect mobilizing change talk.
- ☐ Query reasons for family choices with respect to using skills long term. Promote elaboration.
- ☐ Ask family members to reflect on what they learned in previous weeks and how these lessons can inform the action plan.

Case Example for Mobilizing Module 3: Kim and David

David is an eleventh-grade male who attends advanced classes at a public high school in an affluent suburb of a large Midwestern city. He is actively involved in track and field and works in his school's library twice a week after school. His mother, Kim, is in the midst of a divorce from David's father and reports her own current struggles with anxiety and depression. Throughout treatment, Kim struggled to monitor David's skill use on a daily basis, often feigning her participation in weekly activities. Despite his mother's variable participation, David somewhat consistently practiced new skills of keeping his assignments logged into his smartphone and making a list each day to help him organize homework time.

Discussion: Building a Daily Routine

The therapist can begin the session by discussing the family's experience tracking parent and teen skill practice during the past week. During this conversation, the therapist can begin by asking family members to share their experiences with the tracking assignment—namely, noticing each day whether or not the tasks were completed. As part of this conversation, the family should discuss how accurate they believed their recorded results to be and whether there were any tasks that they were unable to monitor due to insufficient information.

Next, the therapist can ask the parent and teen to share tasks that were completed consistently during the past week. As a part of this conversation, the therapist can affirm the successes of the family and evoke change talk related to the benefits of consistent skill practice. The therapist can also ask the parent and teen to identify tasks on the list that do not yet seem to be habits. The therapist can evoke preparatory change talk by asking the parent and teen to explain why they would like to continue to practice these skills and what they think it would take for them to turn them into habits. The therapist can normalize that some habits take a lot of practice before they can form. Looking ahead, the therapist can elicit how the family thinks life will be different once unformed habits are in place.

Therapeutic Progress

David reported that he used his phone to record his homework every day during the past week and also used a homework list daily. He was pleased to share that he also began practicing his guitar more frequently. Kim expressed that she believed David to be untruthful. She also acknowledged that she did not participate in the home exercise because she felt too much divorce-related stress. During the session Kim demanded David's phone and, upon examination, announced that he had not recorded any assignments on Thursday or Friday. David calmly reminded his mother that he did not have school on Thursday or homework on Friday. The therapist affirmed David's efforts and reflected Kim's difficult state of ambivalence—on the one hand, she may be feeling that her mental health and marital problems need to take priority, and, on the other hand, she really wants to be a supportive parent to David. Together the therapist and the family discussed small, manageable ways for Kim to support David in the present moment. Kim indicated that she would be willing to consider monitoring whether David makes a homework list each night.

Progress Review

This component of the session is described in Chapter 6.

Discussion: Forming an Action Plan

After weeks of practicing new skills one by one, the therapist should guide the family to create an action plan—that is, a plan for moving forward that designates how home will be structured to support skill practice. This plan typically names a handful of responsibilities that the teen must complete before accessing enjoyable activities. Considering the results of the home activity, the teen and parent can be asked to consider what tasks they might want to place on the action plan.

Therapeutic Progress

David states that his priorities are using his phone to keep track of homework assignments and continuing to use lists as a strategy to organize his homework time. They continue their discussion about realistic parental support, and the two agree that David will text his mother a picture of his nightly list once he completes it. Kim agrees that she can text David back with any comments she has on his list, and the therapist uses a scaling question to probe and affirm her level of confidence. Kim indicated that on a scale from 0 to 10, her confidence level sits earnestly at about a 5. When asked what she would need to increase her confidence level slightly, Kim said she would need to be less stressed about her divorce. The therapist considers referring Kim to counseling for her own difficulties.

KEY POINT: Selecting Priority Areas for an Action Plan

When deciding what tasks to place on an action plan, the parent and teen may want to consider:

How many? Putting too many tasks on an action plan can make it overly complicated, creating too many points of failure. Simplicity is key. Typically, using no more than three tasks is recommended.

Link to goals: The parent and teen may prioritize tasks that will help the teen meet his or her engagement module 2 goals.

Observability: If the parent is unable to monitor whether or not the task occurred, it will be hard to maintain a structure that requires responsibilities before enjoyable activities. The parent may land in a situation in which he or she is unsure whether to grant access to enjoyable activities because it is unclear whether responsibilities were completed.

Routine: The action plan contains a section for daily tasks that must be completed before daily enjoyable activities may occur. It also contains a section for less frequently occuring tasks (e.g., a weekly organization check) that should be completed before less frequent enjoyable activities may take place (e.g., weekend activity with friends). The parent and teen should carefully consider under which section of the plan each task falls.

Discussion: How to Structure an Action Plan

The therapist can use EPE (see Chapter 4) to introduce the concept of the action plan, which allows the family to devise a structure for the home environment that reinforces use of new compensatory skills. As part of this conversation, the therapist can elicit from the family any ideas they have already about an action plan for moving forward that would create a daily routine for the skills they would like to practice. One part of this plan is coming up with the routine. A second part is coming up with the structure that supports this routine (i.e., designating how certain enjoyable activities will wait until after responsibilities are complete).

The therapist can refer to Worksheet 7.7, which is an information sheet on creating an action plan. Continuing with EPE, the therapist can guide the family to review each piece of information on the sheet and to provide their reactions. The therapist can emphasize the family members' autonomy in creating an action plan that works best for their unique circumstances.

To conclude this discussion, the therapist can ask permission to begin a collaboratively devised action plan using the tasks prioritized earlier in the session.

In-Session Exercise: Create an Action Plan ✪

The therapist can refer to the action plan template on Worksheet 7.8. To begin the activity, the therapist can encourage the family to consider lessons learned about what kind of home structure best encourages teen skill use. As the therapist guides the family through the action plan template, he or she can continue to evoke mobilizing change talk, asking family members to explain their choices.

As part of contract completion, the therapist and the family can discuss how many weeks they will practice the contract prior to scheduling mobilizing module 4. Depending on the family's level of self-sufficiency, it may be appropriate to wait 1 week or even up to 1 month before holding the next session.

Therapeutic Progress

Usually, action plans (see Figure 7.6 on page 198) should stipulate a structure in which the parent monitors whether all tasks are complete before the teen can participate in enjoyable activities. However, in the case of David, Kim does not yet feel ready to offer this level of involvement because of her personal situation. On the other hand, the level of involvement to which she commits is a step in the right direction for her. In this case the therapist helps the family implement an action plan that feels realistic to their current situation. Because David is in eleventh grade, he can play an active role in his own practice monitoring. The two put their action plan on paper and elaborate that if David has no missing assignments during the week, he will go on a special outing with his mother on Saturdays. The pair expressed

KEY POINTS: Moving from Single-Skill Contracts to an Action Plan

Thus far, all contracts have included only one skill that must be practiced prior to participation in enjoyable activities. However, in many cases, families hope to practice more than one skill simultaneously, and it may be confusing to integrate multiple skills into a working action plan. For example, what happens if the teen completes one task but not another? There is no single best way to organize an action plan; families should be encouraged to consider what they've learned thus far in designing their own personalized plan.

Daily versus Nondaily Tasks

Daily tasks should be linked to enjoyable activities that the teen already does on a daily basis. Less frequent tasks, such as a weekly organization check, should be linked to enjoyable activities the teen does on a less frequent basis (a point system can be helpful in these cases; see skill module 3).

Linking Tasks to Enjoyable Activities

All or nothing. Families may decide to use an all-or-nothing approach, deeming that all skills or responsibilities must occur before enjoyable activities can take place.

   One enjoyable activity per task. Families may decide to designate different enjoyable activities for each task. This option is prone to backfire unless the activities are very distinct from each other. For example, earning evening computer time for writing down homework and evening video game time for completing homework creates a problem when the teen decides the video game time is not important since he already has earned access to the computer. A successful example of this approach might be allowing the teen to use electronics on the car ride for writing in the planner and in the evening for completing homework.

Determining Which Enjoyable Activities Can Be Accessed

Activity menu. Families may decide to allow teens to select one enjoyable activity at a time off of a menu once responsibilities are complete.

   Free access. Families may decide to allow teens to access all enjoyable activities once responsibilities are complete.

Bonuses

Setting weekly or monthly bonuses can be a useful way to acknowledge consistent teen efforts. Adolescents may earn points for each perfect day that are later counted toward a less frequently occurring enjoyable activity (e.g., a special outing). Of course, similar to daily structure, bonus structure should only include enjoyable activities that the teen already does on an intermittent basis (rather than new rewards). Creating a bonus structure is often a way of further enhancing teen motivation to push through boring or difficult tasks.

Part 1: Daily Structure

(A) I will practice the following tasks *daily*:

Put all my homework assignments in my phone and make a list before I start

doing my homework. Finish all my homework.

(B) **Teen list of enjoyable activities that must wait until after daily tasks are complete:** *TV, going online, video games*

(C) **Parent role in reinforcing part (B):** *Text with David to see if he's got his list organized for homework time. When I remember, I'll talk to him about whether he's done it.*

(D) **To promote independence for (A), what parent will *not* do:** *Parent will not yell or become angry if he doesn't do his part.*

Part 2: Weekly Structure (Optional)

(A) **List any tasks that will be completed each week, but not daily. Also list when they will occur.**

Not applicable.

(B) **What enjoyable activity that is not daily must wait until after (A) is complete? Specify if you will use a point system.** *Not applicable.*

(C) **Parent role in reinforcing part (B):** *Not applicable.*

(D) **To promote independence, what parent will *not* do:** *Not applicable.*

Part 3: Bonuses (Optional)

List any bonuses that the teen may earn and how the teen may earn them: *On Saturdays, we will go get coffee together, and David can pick out a new vinyl record at the music store next door if he has no missing assignments during the week according to his online gradebook.*

| _____ | _____ |
| Teen Signature | Parent Signature |

FIGURE 7.6. Sample action plan.

All group sessions begin with a joint homework review from the last session.

Parent Content: Using the subgroup discussion format, parents can discuss their ideas for creating an action plan. Parents can also discuss tasks they believe should be integrated into the action plan, based on the results of the habit-tracking activity. As part of this discussion, parents can review the action plan ideas on Worksheet 7.7 and discuss which might be most useful for their teens.

Teen Content: Teens can also discuss ideas for action plans, reviewing what they like about contracts that they've tried thus far. They can also discuss which skills they would like to turn into habits, referring to the results of the previous week's habit-tracking experiment. The therapist can review Worksheet 7.7 with teens, discussing different ideas for creating an action plan.

Collaborative Content ✪: Parents and teens complete Worksheet 7.8, which asks them to draft an action plan that builds a home structure around the completion of multiple daily and weekly tasks.

FIGURE 7.7. Delivering mobilizing module 3 in a group.

confidence in their plan—particularly because of the text messaging system and an agreement that they remind each other to do their parts. Despite her partial involvement in the action plan, Kim offered the following promising change talk at the end of the session: "I've seen him making progress, and I don't want my personal problems to get in the way of his success."

Home Exercise: Implement an Action Plan

The therapist should direct the parent's and teen's attention to Worksheet 7.9, which contains a progress log for the tasks listed on the action plan. The therapist should discuss with the family how to use the log to monitor how the action plan is going between sessions.

Mobilizing Module 4: Keeping Momentum

Checklist for Mobilizing Module 4

Materials

☐ None

Worksheet

☐ Worksheet 7.10. Next Steps

Topics

☐ Review action plan
☐ Positive changes
☐ Progress on goals

☐ Continuing practice
☐ Advice for new families
☐ Next steps

Key MI Skills

☐ Reframe negative experiences as important learning opportunities.
☐ Affirm parent and teen successes integrating skills into new routines.
☐ Listen for and reflect mobilizing change talk.
☐ Affirm positive changes made during treatment.
☐ Offer autonomy support statements attributing progress to specific actions by the parent and the teen.
☐ Emphasize the difference between life before and after new parent and teen routines.

Case Example for Mobilizing Module 4: Maria and Vinny

Vinny is a 14-year-old eighth-grade student in regular classes at a public school who attended treatment with his mother, Maria. At the beginning of STAND, Vinny articulated goals to remember his homework better, to keep his backpack organized, and to stay out of trouble at school. His mother reported constant reminding and checking during homework time and indicated a desire to offer less assistance to Vinny. Over the course of treatment, the two devised a plan for Vinny to get signatures in his planner from his teachers, who would also write a note if he had any behavior problems in class. The pair came up with an initial plan to allow video games only if Vinny correctly wrote in his planner and had no behavior problems at school. However, Maria decided that the arguments that arose when she asked Vinny to stop playing were too problematic to continue use of this privilege. Instead, she decided video games would only be allowed on the weekends, and the two decided to use the cell phone as an enjoyable activity that he could have access to during the week. In his action plan, Vinny asked for a bonus of being able to spend time at his neighbor's house on Saturdays if he had no behavior problems at school during the week.

Discussion: Review Action Plan

The therapist can begin the session by asking the family to share their experiences implementing the action plan. The therapist can focus the first part of the conversation on aspects of the plan that were successful. During this part of the discussion, the therapist can affirm positive efforts by the parent and the teen—even inconsistent implementation represents attempts to improve the status quo and should be recognized. The therapist can also elicit and reflect mobilizing change talk about steps taken toward creating change, the positive consequences of those steps, and the family members' hopes for the future based on continuation of new habits.

The therapist can also discuss lessons learned during the past week(s) that might inform revision of the action plan. When problems occur with the action plan, the therapist can affirm family efforts and emphasize that progress often occurs slowly when teens and families struggle with attention, EF, or motivation difficulties, which are lifelong challenges that require slow development of compensatory skills. Following a thorough discussion of efforts, the therapist can ask family members what they plan to do with respect to continuing STAND strategies at home after treatment ceases.

Therapeutic Progress

Maria and Vinny were pleased with their consistent implementation of an action plan during the preceding 2 weeks. Maria shared that Vinny recently received a report card that had all A's and B's. Vinny described the new skills he had been practicing and bragged that he had gotten all of his teacher signatures in his planner. His mother added that he had not been in trouble at school since the new plan started. Maria also disclosed that she finally was able to meet with Vinny's school earlier in the week. She said that she dreaded the meeting, expecting to be blamed as a parent for Vinny's misbehavior. Instead, Vinny's teachers had said that he had a lot of potential and that they had noticed that he had lately been working to stay on task in class.

Maria recounted how she had developed a new routine for herself in which she asked Vinny to open his planner and hand her his phone as soon as he got in the car after school. When Vinny had signatures missing from his planner, she sent him back inside the school. The therapist asked Vinny and Maria how they envisioned life would be in a year if they both continued their recent habits. Vinny said he believed he could get straight A's, and his mother said that she hoped his new skills would slowly become automatic over the next year, so that she would no longer need to check his progress or monitor his cell phone to support his academic habits.

Discussion: Positive Changes

For the next portion of mobilizing module 4, the therapist should ask the parent and teen to consider positive changes they think each made during treatment. The parent and teen should consider personal changes, as well as changes noticed in the other person.

Therapeutic Progress

Maria reflected on the personal changes she made during the program and stated that she learned to leave Vinny alone during homework and to be consistent with a structure that requires responsibilities to come before fun. The therapist linked these parental changes to Vinny's improvements. Maria acknowledged that having

> **KEY POINT:** *Discussion of Positive Changes*
>
> The therapist's goal during this session is to elicit mobilizing change talk that links parent and teen efforts to positive outcomes in their lives. Key points of discussion include:
>
> - Emphasizing that changes are of the parent's and teen's personal doing.
> - Affirming all successful efforts—even if there weren't many.
> - Deepening change talk to find its emotional components.
> - Asking parents to identify how their own actions led to improvements for the teen.
> - Discussing why it is important to continue positive changes.
> - Asking family members to identify what it will take to maintain changes long term.
> - What the family members hope will happen in the future if changes continue.

a therapist to support her through the process was an important ingredient in having the courage to try something new. Vinny shared that he felt that his mother was calmer since beginning therapy and was allowing him more space during homework time, which reduced arguments at home.

Discussion: Progress on Goals

Referring to the goals listed in engagement module 2, the therapist can hold a final discussion with the parent and teen on their perceived progress toward each listed goal. This conversation can build on the previous one by talking about where the family hopes to go next in continuing to move toward unmet goals.

If changes in support of the goal have not yet occurred, the therapist can focus on eliciting preparatory change talk regarding desires or ability to make a change in the area. If progress is notable but the goal has not yet been met, the therapist can consider with the family members what steps have been taken in support of the goal, whether the goal is realistic, and what additional steps might be taken to pursue the goal. For example:

THERAPIST: Vinny, the first goal you have on here is keeping track of your homework assignments.

VINNY: I've been writing in my planner every day, so I'd say it's going well.

THERAPIST: It's true, you have been very consistent at using your planner. How did you get to that point?

VINNY: I tried to just focus on getting it done and then it also helped me focus to know that I had to get it done before I could use my cell phone.

THERAPIST: That structure you and Mom came up with played a big part in writing down your homework. What do you think is your next step to turn this practice into a natural habit?

VINNY: My mom needs to trust me more, like not have to check it. In high school next year, I don't really want to go up to the teachers and get their initials.

THERAPIST: You are looking forward to managing your homework a little bit more independently. Mom, what do you need to see to feel comfortable letting him do it without your supervision?

MARIA: I'm not there yet. I know he's made tremendous progress in this area, but it's only been 2 months. I agree with him that maybe when he is in high school we can do things differently, but for now I think he still needs that structure to keep him practicing.

THERAPIST: So you both think the next step is for Vinny to have less supervision—when he's ready. Right now the goal is to keep practicing.

Therapeutic Progress

Vinny examined his goals from the engagement module 2 and commented on each. He noted that he was writing in his planner daily—attributing his success to knowing that his teacher and mother were paying attention to whether he did it or not. He also mentioned feeling more motivated to do his homework—sometimes because of wanting to use his cell phone, but other times because he just wanted to get it over with. Vinny asked his mother if she would trust him to practice the skills without a contract and she hesitated, explaining that she would like to see progress for a few more months before abandoning the structure that seemed to be helping. The two decided to continue implementing the action plan but to shift to a less structured plan when Vinny began high school the following year.

Discussion: Continuing Practice

The therapist can hold a conversation about what the parent and teen learned about the process of forming new habits. The therapist can elicit from the parent and teen ideas about how they were able to form new habits over the course of treatment. As part of this conversation, the therapist can ask the family members to discuss what they think they would do if they wanted to form a new habit and what they think they would do if an old habit started to fade. EPE (see Chapter 4) can be used to interchange family ideas with key points about habit formation that the therapist can offer as ideas other families have shared in the past.

Therapeutic Progress

Looking back, Vinny was able to identify wanting to please his teachers and his mother as a primary reason for practicing his new skills. He also mentioned that

> ### KEY POINT: Maintaining New Habits
>
> The concept of how to form and maintain new habits is one of the critical pieces of knowledge that families can glean from treatment. Each family is unique, and so the process of habit formation may look different for each teen and parent. Some key considerations to discuss with families include:
>
> **Daily practice.** Daily practice is typically required to form lasting habits.
>
> **Structure helps.** Daily practice is much more likely to occur with good structure at home—namely one that puts skill practice before fun activities.
>
> **Noticing benefits.** Once a new skill is regularly practiced, discussions with the teen about natural benefits of using the new skill can help the teen build additional motivation to continue practice.
>
> **Phasing out parent support.** Once the habit appears to occur on a regular basis, the parent and teen can discuss whether the parent can reduce her or his role in supporting skill use. Removing formal action plans or contracts allows the family to observe whether the teen is capable of maintaining the habit without parental support.

previously he saw himself as a bad student and didn't believe that he could be successful in school. Vinny expressed a desire to reach out to his teachers and mother for support if he found his motivation waning. His mother said it worked well for her to check the planner as soon as she picked him up from school—a consistent event that happened the same way for her each day.

Discussion: Advice for New Families

As the session comes to a close, the therapist can prompt the parent and the teen to consider pieces of advice they would give to new families who are just starting the program. The parent can be prompted to offer advice to other parents and the teen to other teens. The therapist can reflect parent and teen advice statements in ways that deepen their meaning and explore their reasons. For example:

THERAPIST: Mom, I wonder what advice you might have for a new parent who is just starting this program with his or her teen.

MARIA: To stay consistent. The plans we are supposed to do at home are hard to remember, especially when things get busy. We didn't always do them, but when we did, it was worth it. When I took the time to do my part, he always did his.

THERAPIST: A few useful pieces of advice in there. Most of all, to give attention to the home practice—that was useful to you.

MARIA: Yes, it helped me see with my own eyes how things could be different if we changed the structure at home. When we finally made a good plan, I was more relaxed because everyone was on the same page.

THERAPIST: You would tell parents that if they put in the time to do the work at home, they will feel more relaxed in the end and that their teen will probably put in more work, too.

MARIA: I would.

THERAPIST: How has that relaxation benefited you personally?

MARIA: I am nagging less because I can trust the new structure. I don't have to think as much about whether to punish him if he misbehaves. We already have a plan in place that everyone knows.

THERAPIST: You have more confidence in your parenting choices because you've thought through them and tested them out.

Therapeutic Progress

Maria's advice to other parents is to do the home exercises. She states that she did not always do them at first and that changes did not begin to occur until she decided to start monitoring and seriously implementing the cell phone rule. She reflected that when she took the time to do her part, Vinny always took the time to do his. Maria added that she feels more relaxed when relying on rules rather than reasoning to encourage Vinny to be responsible each day. Vinny stated that his advice to a new teen in the program is to try hard, believe in yourself, and use your planner.

Next Steps ✪

To close the session, the therapist can refer to Worksheet 7.10 and ask the parents and teen to consider concrete next steps that they would like to make in the next month to maintain steady progress. The parent and teen can be asked to write down these next steps and can be encouraged to post the next steps in a place where they can remember them. In addition, the parent and teen can write at the bottom of the page their personal reasons for wanting to follow the next steps. To close the activity, the parent and teen can be asked a future-oriented question about where they hope they will be next year if they continue their progress.

Therapeutic Progress

Vinny makes a verbal commitment to continuing to use his planner, approaching teachers to sign the planner, and behaving well in class. Maria expresses that she intends to continue the action plan for the rest of the year. The therapist reflects her worries that removing this structure too soon could disrupt Vinny's progress. Maria states that she feels in better control with the new structure in place. The therapist reflects the pair's shared investment in Vinny's academic success and affirms their hard work during treatment.

All group sessions begin with a joint home activity review from the last session.

Parent Content: Using the subgroup discussion format, parents can discuss progress over the course of treatment, their use of the action plan, ideas for continuing progress, next steps, and their advice for future families.

Teen Content: Similarly, the therapist can facilitate discussions with teens that cover their progress, their impressions of the contract used during the last week, and any next steps they think they should take to continue progress. Teens can write letters to future teens in the program and share these letters collaboratively with their groupmates.

Collaborative Content ○: Parents and teens complete **Worksheet 7.10**, which asks them to discuss their expectations for future skill use following the conclusion of the program.

FIGURE 7.8. Delivering mobilizing module 4 in a group.

Whether to Terminate after Mobilizing Module 4

If the treatment process occurs in a measured fashion, with engagement and skill modules repeated as needed, most families seem ready to terminate treatment at mobilizing module 4. If families would benefit from additional sessions, additional sessions can be delivered using the problem-solving format of skill module 7 or any module that seems appropriate (see Chapter 2). At the end of mobilizing module 4, the therapist and the families should discuss expectations for future contact, including the possibility of and time frame for continued sessions.

What new skills do the parent and teen hope to continue practicing?

Which aspects of these new skills occur in the school setting?

How can information about practice of skills at school help the parent and teen build accountability?

What kinds of supports or communication do you hope to obtain from the school in support of the efforts described above?

Initially Engaging School Staff	Maintaining School Staff Engagement
• Remind yourself of positive things the teacher has done. • Praise and thank teachers for their efforts. • Recognize concerns noted by the teacher. • Ask teachers what you can do to facilitate home–school communication. • Listen to and summarize teacher suggestions. • Politely suggest modifications to teacher suggestions as needed. • Allow teachers to contribute ideas to the conversation. • Agree to requests made by teachers. • Ask teachers the best way to contact them. • Give teachers your contact information and encourage them to contact you. • Find ways to show genuine appreciation to teachers. • Continue to thank teachers throughout the year when they provide consistent efforts.	• Approach teachers from a problem-solving perspective. • Address a problem as soon as it begins. • Ask teachers if everything is all right when their support seems to drop off. • Provide teachers with gentle prompts or reminders. • Ask teachers how you can help them. • Ask teachers what they think you can do differently. • Let teachers know how much their previous efforts have been helpful. • Point out evidence of the teen's improvement to make sure they notice.

1. Points the teen would like to make during this conversation:

2. Points the parent would like to make during this conversation:

3. What are some positive things you can say to the school staff member?

4. What questions would the teen like to ask the teacher?

5. What questions would the parent like to ask the teacher?

6. What strategies would be particularly helpful to remember when working with the school staff member?

1. What are the teen's next steps to engage school staff in supporting skill practice?

2. What can the teen do in the next week?

3. What are the parent's next steps to engage school staff in supporting the parent's skill practice?

4. What can the parent do in the next week?

Place strategies that you have practiced in the toolbox. Circle ones that you would like to turn into an automatic habit.

TEEN TOOLBOX

PARENT TOOLBOX

WORKSHEET 7.6. Building a Daily Routine

1. Look at your toolbox. Below, write down skills that you would like to build into your daily routine.

2. Add any responsibilities at home that you would like to build into a daily routine.

Track these tasks on a daily basis for the next week.

Mark a **Y** if the task occurred successfully.
Mark an **N** if the task did not occur or was incomplete.
Mark a **?** if the parent and teen are unsure whether the task occurred.

When will the parent and teen find time to complete this sheet each day? _____

	Day 1	Day 2	Day 3	Day 4	Day 5	Day 6	Day 7	Day 8
Teen Morning Tasks								
Teen School Tasks								
Teen Evening Tasks								
Parent Tasks								

Daily versus Nondaily Tasks

- Daily tasks can go on part 1 of action plan

AND

- Tasks that might occur once or twice a week can go on part 2 of action plan.

Daily versus Nondaily Enjoyable Activities

- Enjoyable activities that typically occur daily should be linked to daily tasks

AND

- Enjoyable activities that typically occur less than daily should be linked to nondaily tasks

Linking Tasks to Enjoyable Activities

- You can make all enjoyable activities wait until after all tasks are complete

OR

- You can grant a separate enjoyable activity for each task that is completed (but be careful that each enjoyable activity does not overlap or compete with each other).

Determining Which Enjoyable Activities Can Be Accessed

- You can use an activity menu that lists all enjoyable activities and the teen can select one enjoyable activity off of the menu once tasks are complete

OR

- You can grant free access to any and all enjoyable activities once tasks are complete.

Bonuses

- You can include weekly or monthly bonuses for consistently following the action plan.
- Teens can earn points toward bonuses.
- Once the teen accrues enough points, a special activity can be offered.
- This activity can help build teen motivation to perform tasks that are especially hard to remember or complete.

Part 1: Daily Structure

(A) I will practice the following tasks *daily*:

_____

_____

_____

(B) Teen list of enjoyable activities that must wait until after daily tasks are complete:

(C) Parent role in reinforcing part (B):

(D) To promote independence for (A), what parent will *not* do:

Part 2: Weekly Structure (Optional)

(A) List any tasks that will be completed each week, but not daily. Also list when they will occur.

_____

_____

(B) What enjoyable activity that is *not daily* must wait until after (A) is complete? Specify if you will use a point system.

(C) Parent role in reinforcing part (B):

(D) To promote independence, what parent will *not* do:

Part 3: Bonuses (Optional)

List any bonuses that the teen may earn and how the teen may earn them:

_____   _____
Teen Signature   Parent Signature

WORKSHEET 7.9. Action Plan Log

Week: _____	M	T	W	Th	F	Weekly Bonus?
Teen Skill 1:						
Teen Skill 2:						Y N
Teen Skill 3:						
Activities Earned?	Y N	Y N	Y N	Y N	Y N	
Week: _____ Goals	M	T	W	Th	F	Weekly Bonus?
Teen Skill 1:						
Teen Skill 2:						Y N
Teen Skill 3:						
Activities Earned?	Y N	Y N	Y N	Y N	Y N	
Week: _____ Goals	M	T	W	Th	F	Weekly Bonus?
Teen Skill 1:						
Teen Skill 2:						Y N
Teen Skill 3:						
Activities Earned?	Y N	Y N	Y N	Y N	Y N	

In the next month, what steps does the teen hope to make to continue progress toward goals?

In the next month, what steps does the parent hope to make to continue progress toward goals?

What are the teen's personal reasons for wanting to take these steps?

What are the parent's personal reasons for wanting to take these steps?

Where will this page be posted to serve as a reminder?

CHAPTER 8

Clinical Advice

T his chapter shares a range of suggestions for working with families of teens with attention, EF, and motivation deficits. Common challenges are highlighted, along with potential strategies to address them.

Disengagement

Adolescent Nonparticipation in Discussions

It is not surprising that teens who fail to participate actively in school may also fail to participate in therapy. Nonparticipation may occur for several reasons. Some teens are accustomed to parents speaking for them. Other teens expect high levels of assistance with daily tasks, finding an emphasis on autonomy to be uncomfortable at first. Yet other teens may be shy, unsure of what to say, or uninterested in participating.

Much of STAND is designed to reduce oppositional behavior by valuing the teen's voice and respecting the teen's desired level of participation. However, some teens' refusal to participate in treatment takes the form of ignoring the parent or therapist. In our experience, this defiance is typically directed more toward the parent than the therapist. However, parent-directed anger can result in refusal to speak during session.

Recommended Strategies for Addressing Adolescent Nonparticipation

FIRST STEPS

- Assess the nature of teen reluctance and tailor interactions accordingly.
- Ask open-ended questions to elicit information from the teen.

- Affirm the teen for small contributions to therapy discussions.
- Emphasize that the teen is an important participant in treatment

NEXT STEPS

- Pause and wait for the teen's answers—even when it creates elongated silence.
- Prevent the parent from answering for the teen.
- Assert a desire to hear the teen's viewpoint.
- Communicate respect for the teen's feelings.
- If a teen actively refuses to participate, clarify that he or she is not required to contribute to discussions.
- Invite an actively refusing teen to join the conversation whenever he or she feels like it.

Example

THERAPIST: Alex, I get the sense that you aren't happy about being here today.

ALEX: Nope.

THERAPIST: It wasn't your choice.

ALEX: My mom made me come here.

THERAPIST: Thanks for being honest, Alex. You certainly don't have to participate in any parts of this meeting that you don't want to. It's your choice if you decide to join the conversation.

ALEX: I know.

THERAPIST: If it's OK with you, I'm going to talk with Mom a little bit about how the week went. I hope you'll chime in if you have an opinion because you are the most important person here.

Parent Displacement of Blame

Some parents fail to acknowledge their contribution to the teen's difficulties, instead blaming the teen for problems. Displacement of blame can lead parents to participate minimally in therapy activities. Furthermore, parents who believe therapy should be teen-directed may develop distaste for a parent–teen collaborative approach because it emphasizes parental involvement.

Recommended Strategies for Addressing Parent Displacement of Blame

FIRST STEPS

- Frame treatment as training the adolescent to complete responsibilities independently.
- Frame home activities as an experiment, rather than a permanent change.

- Affirm all parental efforts and reflect change talk about the benefits of home practice.

NEXT STEPS

- Elicit change talk from the parent about the benefits of new parenting strategies.
- Link parental actions to teen functioning.
- Elicit change talk from the parent about the importance of teen success.
- Link teen success to the parent's priorities.

Failure to Practice at Home

Families may repeatedly fail to complete home activities. Treatment is likely to be unsuccessful without skill practice at home. When this happens, it is typically a function of poor parental engagement.

Recommended Strategies for Addressing Failure to Practice at Home

FIRST STEPS

- Affirm all positive parental efforts during the past week—even if they were small.
- Elicit the benefits of small steps taken.
- Elicit change talk that links parental actions to teen improvements.
- Ask family whether they would like to retry incomplete home activities.
- Allow opportunities to complete brief home activities prior to continuing the current session.
- Allow family to decide if they will try daily skill practice again over the next week.

NEXT STEPS

- Use the readiness ruler to probe interest when planning subsequent home exercises.
- Suggest realistic home activities that encourage small steps toward success.
- Brainstorm strategies to help the parent remember to practice at home.
- Consider repeating engagement modules to build investment.
- Hold an honest conversation with the family about their interest in continuing treatment

Session Management

Teen Refusal to Sign a Contract

In some cases, a teen may refuse to sign a contract because he or she is upset or angry about parental attempts to set limits on his or her freedoms.

Recommended Strategies for Addressing Teen Refusal

FIRST STEPS

- Emphasize the teen's autonomy in treatment.
- Ask the teen to share his or her concerns.
- Reflect without judgment unreasonable or counterproductive demands by the teen.
- Ask the family how they want to proceed.
- Emphasize the experimental nature of home activities.

NEXT STEPS

- Suggest that the teen take notes on all problems he or she notices with a contract during the upcoming week.
- Allow the parent to proceed without the input of the teen if the teen's behavior seems unreasonable.
- Suggest that the parent still practice reinforcing structure at home, emphasizing that the adolescent has the choice of whether or not to practice the skills each day.

Example

COLTON: I'm not signing this. It isn't fair.

THERAPIST: You certainly shouldn't sign a contract you aren't comfortable with. Talk me through your concerns.

COLTON: I like to play video games after school. It's the only way I can relax after having to work all day. If I don't get time to relax, then I won't be able to focus on my homework.

PARENT: Once you start playing video games you refuse to stop. Then I end up fighting with you over it. This structure makes a lot more sense. Finish your homework and you can play as long as you want to.

COLTON: No way. This isn't fair at all. You are punishing me and I haven't done anything wrong.

THERAPIST: You both agree it's important to get homework done. Colton, you don't think it's fair for video games to wait until after homework because you like to play right after school. Mom, you feel pretty strongly that relaxation time needs to come after homework.

COLTON: Everything is fine the way it is. We don't need to make these changes.

THERAPIST: It's possible that you don't need to make a change. I guess we'd need to try it out to know for sure. How open would you be to trying this out for 1 week? Just as an experiment. You could come back and tell us if it worked or not.

COLTON: If it's just 1 week. I'll think about it. But I'm not ready to agree yet.

THERAPIST: So where does this leave us?

COLTON: I'm going to think about it.

THERAPIST: It's mature that you are willing to give this some consideration, Colton. I understand not wanting to commit until you've given it some thought.

COLTON: We'll see.

THERAPIST: You and Mom are certainly welcome to sign it later when you have had a chance to think.

PARENT: Why don't we talk about it again tomorrow?

THERAPIST: Colton, it's really up to you, but if you decide you don't want to participate this week, would it be OK for Mom to still practice her part?

COLTON: What do you mean?

THERAPIST: Well, Mom may want an opportunity to practice with her new skills at home. She may want to practice monitoring whether you do your homework.

COLTON: I don't care if she asks to see my homework.

THERAPIST: You're willing to let her see your homework. She may also be interested in practicing the skill of setting limits on video game time. Parents sometimes need practice at that part, too.

COLTON: You mean take video games away from me?

THERAPIST: It's really up to Mom what kind of approach she wants to practice.

PARENT: Let's talk about this tomorrow. I think we can revisit this when everyone is calmer.

Arriving to Session Angry

In some cases, an adolescent or parent may come to session already angry about something that happened earlier in the day. This may distract from the intended purpose of the session.

Recommended Strategies for Addressing Arriving to Session Angry

FIRST STEPS

- Use engagement module 3 skills to work through the challenging situation.

NEXT STEPS

- Postpone the session until the parent and teen are calmer.

Parent–Teen Conflict

When parent–teen conflict is repeatedly high during sessions, it may prevent the therapist from covering session material.

Recommended Strategies for Addressing Parent–Teen Conflict

FIRST STEPS

- Use engagement module 3 skills to work through the challenging situation.
- Moderate discussions by using reflections that summarize parent and teen concerns and move the conversation forward.

NEXT STEPS

- Hold an honest discussion with the family about their level of conflict in session.
- Use an object that symbolizes permission to talk (e.g., a talking stone).
- Place time limits on parent and teen comments.
- Allow family members to decide if they would like to implement session rules.

Example

THERAPIST: Is it OK if I share something that has been challenging to me as a therapist?

PARENT: Sure.

THERAPIST: I'm really enjoying working with your family, and I'm struggling a little bit because I haven't been able to get through all of our material because of the arguments that come up during our meetings.

PARENT: I know. We just are very stressed right now.

THERAPIST: It's really up to you how we proceed. But I thought I'd bring this issue up. I guess I might have a few suggestions, if you are interested.

PARENT: Yes, of course.

THERAPIST: Maybe we can go back to the communication skills we practiced a few weeks ago. I wonder if spending more time on them might help us have calmer sessions?

PARENT: I think that sounds OK.

THERAPIST: I want to respect your right to talk about issues that are important to you, and I also worry that we won't be able to get to everything you want to work on if we don't try a new approach.

PARENT: We appreciate that.

THERAPIST: Do you have any advice for me as your therapist?

Interparental Discord

When two parents attend STAND, sessions may be overtaken by interparental disagreements, removing focus from the teen.

Recommended Strategies for Addressing Interparental Discord

FIRST STEPS

- Redirect parental disagreements to refocus treatment on the teen.

NEXT STEPS

- Tell parents that treatment is often more equitable and productive when just one parent participates because it levels the playing field for the teen.
- Hold an honest conversation with the parents about the benefits and disadvantages of their mutual participation.

Parental Interference

Excessive Helping and Reminding

Some parents struggle to surrender the personal assistant role discussed in engagement module 1. Teens will not learn to initiate skill use independently if parents rely on reminders and helping to prompt teen practice. In these cases, teens lose the opportunity to develop an independent habit. Instead, they continue to rely on the parent for prompts, and parental complaints about dependence continue.

Recommended Strategies for Addressing Parental Interference

FIRST STEPS

- Specify in weekly contracts what the parent will do to promote independence (e.g., refraining from reminders and helping).

NEXT STEPS

- Reflect change talk that strengthens parental goals for increasing teen autonomy or reducing helping behaviors.
- Ask open-ended questions during home activity reviews that probe the parent's level of assistance during the past week.

Parental Disorganization

Parents of teens with attention, EF, and motivation problems often struggle with similar difficulties. These deficits can interfere with setting, monitoring, and reinforcing appropriate structure at home.

Recommended Strategies for Addressing Parental Disorganization

FIRST STEPS

- Make details of parental involvement explicit in contracts.
- Discuss organization strategies to help the parent complete home activities (e.g., phone reminders, schedules, organizing materials).
- Affirm parent efforts to stay organized.

NEXT STEPS

- Discuss parental efforts to stay organized during progress reviews.
- Link improved parental organization habits to improved teen functioning.

Philosophical Differences

Some parents dislike the idea of a home structure that requires the teen to complete responsibilities before participating in enjoyable activities. These parents may state that the teen should not be rewarded for something he or she is expected to do or that privilege removal does not work.

Recommended Strategies for Addressing Philosophical Differences

FIRST STEPS

- Differentiate between structure that puts responsibilities first and reward/privilege removal systems.
- Emphasize that new rewards are not to be introduced into the home routine.
- Acknowledge that not all strategies work for every family.

NEXT STEPS

- Use the readiness ruler to query whether the family would be willing to try out a new structure for the next week.
- Elicit change talk about the benefits of home structure during home activity review.

Parental Fear of Limit Setting

Some parents do not restrict access to fun activities—even when the teen has not done his or her part. They may avoid placing limits on the teen to prevent conflict.

Recommended Strategies for Addressing Fear of Limit Setting

FIRST STEPS

- Ask questions during home exercise review about the parent's ability to withhold enjoyable activities when the teen had not yet earned them.
- Discuss parental reasons for not restricting access to enjoyable activities.

- Empathically reflect ambivalence about placing limits on the teen, eliciting change talk about the benefits of this strategy.
- Affirm small efforts toward limit setting.

NEXT STEPS

- Hold a one-on-one meeting with the parent to role-play and practice restricting access to enjoyable activities.
- Use EPE to make the parent aware that conflict with the teen can temporarily escalate if he or she is not used to receiving limits on freedom. Parental consistency with limit setting is the way out of this temporary conflict.
- Respect a parent's decision to avoid stress at home by not placing limits on the teen if the parent believes it is in the family's best interest.

Parental Insistence on Using Tangible Rewards

Instead of creating natural home structure that promotes skill practice, some parents prefer to use tangible rewards to incentivize success, such as money or food. Using a tangible rewards system is not as powerful as harnessing natural contingencies in the teen's daily environment.

Recommended Strategies for Addressing Insistence on Tangible Rewards

FIRST STEPS

- Clarify with parents that home structure aims to use natural contingencies in the teen's daily environment.
- With permission, explain that other families often find that tangible rewards are not as powerful or long-lasting as restructuring the natural environment.
- Ask the family if they would be willing to try a natural consequence–based home structure for 1 week.

NEXT STEPS

- Allow families to try out a tangible rewards system for 1 week.
- During home activity review, discuss challenges to using a rewards-based approach.
- During home activity review, elicit change talk about the benefits of using a structure that engages natural consequences.

Low Parental Autonomy

Some parents frequently seek out the therapist's advice, seem uncomfortable making their own parenting decisions, and present progress as overly positive to please the therapist. Parents are unlikely to maintain changes after therapy ceases if they do not develop skills and parenting autonomy during treatment.

Recommended Strategies for Addressing Low Parental Autonomy

FIRST STEPS

- Emphasize the parent's autonomy in treatment by making statements about his or her expertise as a parent.
- Affirm parental decision making and efforts.
- Limit advice giving by insisting that the parent is in the best position to know what's best.
- Normalize challenges and struggles during therapy to communicate that it is OK to be honest about difficulties.
- Accept small admissions of difficulty with empathy and affirm the parent's honesty.

NEXT STEPS

- Offer more than one piece of advice and let the parent choose between the two options.
- Hold a private conversation with the parent if it appears that he or she is unwilling to discuss certain topics in front of the teen.

Troubleshooting Home Structure

No Time for Evening Enjoyable Activities

Contingent home structure is most effective when the teen gains immediate access to enjoyable activities once responsibilities are complete. However, the structure of some family schedules is prohibitive of chaining activities in this way.

*Recommended Strategies for Addressing Having No Time
for Enjoyable Evening Activities*

FIRST STEPS

- Explore restructuring the teen's schedule.
- Consider whether extracurricular activities leave the teen with insufficient daily relaxation time.

NEXT STEPS

- Explore earning access to enjoyable activities that do not occur immediately but are salient to the teen.
- Consider enjoyable activities that are not immediate, such as sleeping later in the morning, preferred transportation to school, access to electronics the next day, or not having to perform a chore.

- Consider a secondary reinforcer, such as points toward a weekend activity, using a get-out-of-a-chore-free card, or a tangible reinforcer.

Unsuccessful Home Exercises

Some teens do not use daily skills as designated in the contract and do not appear to be motivated by access to enjoyable activities. Others show effort toward following a contract but are unsuccessful at completing responsibilities. The therapist's first job is to understand why the teen is not responding to the contract. There are many possibilities. The most common are outlined in Table 8.1 on pages 228–229, along with possible modifications to the home structure to address the problem.

Removing Structure Too Early

Some parents may be encouraged by early success and prematurely remove explicit home structure that supports skill practice. They may not inform the therapist that they have ceased monitoring and reinforcement. As a result, the teen's functioning may return to pretreatment levels, and the parent may conclude that therapy was unsuccessful.

Recommended Strategies for Addressing Removing Structure Too Early

FIRST STEPS

- Continue to ask open-ended questions about the parent's role in providing home structure—even after mastery has been demonstrated.
- Use mobilizing module 2 as an opportunity to assess how the teen self-manages skill practice without explicit home structure in place.
- Encourage the parent to be a detective and conduct an experiment to see how the teen responds without structure before permanently removing supports.

NEXT STEPS

- Build parental expectation that progress can be slow and that efforts to increase teen independence should be gradual.
- Suggest that structure be gradually reduced to provide parents with an opportunity to decrease involvement.
- Instead of reducing structure, increase the teen's management of his or her own structure. This can include having the parent intermittently check in with the teen.
- A contract can state that if the teen does not fairly self-manage structure, the parent will resume her or his involvement.

TABLE 8.1. Strategies for Addressing Unsuccessful Home Exercises

Issue	What you might notice	Suggested modifications
Expectations are too difficult for the teen.	Teen does not practice skills. Teen may unrealistically expect skill mastery right away. If teen does not believe he or she can be successful, he or she may see no reason to put in the effort.	Discuss whether expectations are realistic prior to implementing a plan at home. To set appropriate expectations, collect data on teen's current ability to perform the skill. Consider only practicing one skill at a time or practicing approximations of skills, adding components one at a time (e.g., start with teen just bringing home his or her planner).
Teen appears uninterested in enjoyable activities.	Some parents impose convenient activities on the teen, rather than ones he or she most enjoys. Other times, the teen still accesses enjoyable activities (sometimes secretly), even though he or she has not completed responsibilities.	Discuss enthusiasm for enjoyable activities listed in the contract. If interest is low, consider modifications to the plan. Seek a clear contrast between the environments before and after tasks are complete. Encourage the parent to carefully monitor teen access to enjoyable activities.
Inconsistent parent monitoring and reinforcement of structure.	Teen is unmotivated to practice because parent does not enforce structure. Teen learns that efforts are not acknowledged and plans made in session are not taken seriously.	If parental inconsistency is suspected, initiate a discussion about parent efforts to reinforce teen skill practice during the past week. MI can be used to strengthen the perceived benefits of implementing structure. A more realistic contract can be devised if the parent needs smaller steps.
Designated enjoyable activities are unrealistic to provide.	Families may designate enjoyable activities that cannot occur regularly because they are expensive, time intensive, or require participation from others who may not be available.	Use scaling questions to query how realistic it would be for the teen to access designated enjoyable activities on a daily basis. Frame unsuccessful contracts as lessons to inform future home structure.
Parent inability to monitor skill use.	Parents may be unable to obtain evidence that a skill was practiced. They may be unsure of whether the teen has earned access to enjoyable activities.	Encourage parents to notice what they can and cannot monitor successfully. Collaborate with teachers to monitor skill use at school. Engage another adult to supervise homework if the parent cannot do so. Choose a different skill to monitor that still helps with the problem. Remove skills that cannot be monitored from contracts.

(continued)

TABLE 8.1. *(continued)*

Issue	What you might notice	Suggested modifications
Logistical difficulties to restricting electronics access.	Parents may complain that they cannot restrict the teen's access to electronics, typically because he or she needs a device to complete schoolwork.	Parental controls can be used to restrict the teen's access to certain websites. The parent can ask the teen to complete online learning in a public room of the house. The parent can implement a consequence for accessing electronics prematurely. Video game controllers, computer mice, and devices can be locked away. Internet access can be password protected. The parent can perform random checks during online learning or review browser history to monitor the teen's computer use.
Teen loses interest in practicing skills.	Teen successfully practices skills for a few weeks and then stops. Teens may initially practice to please the therapist, obtain parental attention, or try something novel. These reasons may no longer be salient midway through treatment.	The parent may not be implementing home structure consistently, reducing teen response once novelty wears off. The parent may not be setting limits on the teen, which may be a new issue now that the teen no longer earns enjoyable activities every day. A teen's interests can change, which can often be remedied by an activity menu (see Chapter 7).

Additional Interfering Factors

Interference from Comorbidities

What seems like low effort may instead be a by-product of something other than a motivation problem—such as teen depression, sleep problems, or anxiety. For example, teens with high levels of anxiety may struggle to complete homework in a timely manner due to fear of producing imperfect work. In these cases, the teen should be referred for anxiety treatment aimed at reducing perfectionistic behavior. Teens with sleep problems may not complete work because they are too tired or may not be prepared for school in the morning because they have trouble waking up.

Recommended Strategies for Addressing Interference from Comorbidities

FIRST STEPS
- Refer the teen for additional assessment to determine the nature of interfering problems.
- Use this information to decide whether to integrate additional treatment components into STAND, suspend STAND to address comorbidities first, refer to a different provider, or to address comorbidities afterward.

NEXT STEPS

- If treatment proceeds, continue to asses the impact of comorbid symptoms on treatment progress.

Need for Educational Accommodations

It is possible that the teen's educational environment is inappropriate for his or her level of functioning, making it difficult to meet minimal expectations for academic success. This possibility is particularly likely when the student has a comorbid learning disorder that makes understanding concepts difficult or if the student has a particularly slow processing speed that makes it unrealistic for him or her to complete a typical homework load within a reasonable amount of time.

Recommended Strategies for Addressing the Need for Educational Accommodations

FIRST STEPS

- Refer the family for appropriate psychoeducational testing.
- Review the teen's IEP or 504 plan with the family.
- Provide the parent with psychoeducational materials about available accommodations in schools.
- Provide the parent with psychoeducational materials about initiating or modifying IEP or 504 plans to obtain appropriate accommodations.

NEXT STEPS

- Encourage the parent to reach out to school staff to discuss the teen's educational supports.
- Coach the parent to give objective examples of how the student's deficits interfere with his or her ability to complete assigned work appropriately.

Overly Demanding Academic Environments

It is also common for teens with high intelligence who struggle with EF or attention problems to test into rigorous gifted or advanced classes that tax the teen's cognitive load. Although acceptance into these programs may be exciting, and the teen may be capable of learning at an advanced level, he or she may not yet possess the skills needed to manage high workloads and complex academic assignments. In these cases, the family should consider whether the student's advanced placement is interfering with the teen's well-being.

*Recommended Strategies for Addressing Overly Demanding
Academic Environments*

FIRST STEPS

- Adopt equipoise in discussing the teen's academic environment—this issue is typically a personal choice for the family to make.
- Encourage the parent and teen to explore a decisional balance—the pros and cons of remaining in the academic environment.

NEXT STEPS

- Link the academic environment to the parent's and teen's treatment goals and hopes for the future.
- If the family decides to make a change, help the parent and teen explore alternative placements.

Termination

STAND is designed as a springboard for families to begin healthy habit development and identify how to structure the home environment to support teen success. Some families may insist that they are not yet ready for termination or may describe a sudden decline in functioning during the last sessions.

Recommended Strategies for Addressing Hesitance to Terminate

FIRST STEPS

- Communicate faith in the family to independently continue skill practice.
- Outline specific plans for continuing skill use.
- Discuss what to do if functioning deteriorates.
- Normalize ups and downs.

NEXT STEPS

- Schedule a booster session after completing all modules.
- Transition the family to a different kind of treatment that addresses difficulties outside the scope of STAND.

References

Barkley, R. A. (Ed.). (2014). *Attention-deficit hyperactivity disorder: A handbook for diagnosis and treatment* (4th ed.). New York: Guilford Press.

Barkley, R. A., Murphy, K. R., & Fischer, M. (2008). *ADHD in adults: What the science says.* New York: Guilford Press.

Brannan, A. M., Heflinger, C. A., & Bickman, L. (1997). The caregiver strain questionnaire measuring the impact on the family of living with a child with serious emotional disturbance. *Journal of Emotional and Behavioral Disorders, 5*(4), 212–222.

Casey, B. J., Jones, R. M., & Hare, T. A. (2008). The adolescent brain. *Annals of the New York Academy of Sciences, 1124*(1), 111–126.

Castellanos, F. X., Sonuga-Barke, E. J., Milham, M. P., & Tannock, R. (2006). Characterizing cognition in ADHD: Beyond executive dysfunction. *Trends in Cognitive Sciences, 10*(3), 117–123.

Clare, S., Helps, S., & Sonuga-Barke, E. J. (2010). The Quick Delay Questionnaire: A measure of delay aversion and discounting in adults. *ADHD Attention Deficit and Hyperactivity Disorders, 2*(1), 43–48.

Cunningham, C. E. (2006). COPE: Large-group, community-based, family-centered parent training. In R. A. Barkley, *Attention-deficit hyperactivity disorder: A handbook for diagnosis and treatment* (3rd ed., pp. 480–498). New York: Guilford Press.

Eccles, J. S. (2004). Schools, academic motivation, and stage–environment fit. In R. M. Lerner & L. Steinberg (Eds.), *Handbook of adolescent psychology* (2nd ed., pp. 125–153). Hoboken, NJ: Wiley.

Edwards, G., Barkley, R. A., Laneri, M., Fletcher, K., & Metevia, L. (2001). Parent–adolescent conflict in teenagers with ADHD and ODD. *Journal of Abnormal Child Psychology, 29*(6), 557–572.

Evans, S. W., Schultz, B. K., DeMars, C. E., & Davis, H. (2011). Effectiveness of the challenging horizons after-school program for young adolescents with ADHD. *Behavior Therapy, 42*(3), 462–474.

Forgatch, M. S., & Patterson, G. R. (1989). *Parents and adolescents living together: Part 2. Family problem solving.* Eugene, OR: Castalia.

Gray, S. A., Chaban, P., Martinussen, R., Goldberg, R., Gotlieb, H., Kronitz, R., et al. (2012). Effects of a computerized working memory training program on working memory, attention, and academics in adolescents with severe LD and comorbid ADHD: A randomized controlled trial. *Journal of Child Psychology and Psychiatry, 53*(12), 1277–1284.

Greenhill, L., Pliszka, S., Dulcan, M., Bernet, W., Arnold, V., Beitchman, J., et al. (2002). Practice parameter for the use of stimulant medications in the treatment of children, adolescents, and adults. *Journal of the American Academy of Child and Adolescent Psychiatry, 41*(2, Suppl.), 26S–49S.

Langberg, J. M., Epstein, J. N., Becker, S. P., Girio-Herrera, E., & Vaughn, A. J. (2012). Evaluation of the Homework, Organization, and Planning Skills (HOPS) intervention for middle school students with ADHD as implemented by school mental health providers. *School Psychology Review, 41*(3), 342.

Miller, W. R., & Rollnick, S. (2013). *Motivational interviewing: Helping people change* (3rd ed.). New York: Guilford Press.

Molina, B. S., Hinshaw, S. P., Swanson, J. M., Arnold, L. E., Vitiello, B., Jensen, P. S., et al. (2009). The MTA at 8 years: Prospective follow-up of children treated for combined-type ADHD in a multisite study. *Journal of the American Academy of Child and Adolescent Psychiatry, 48*(5), 484–500.

Moyers, T. B., Manuel, J. K., & Ernst, D. (2014). *Motivational interviewing treatment integrity coding manual 4.1.* Unpublished manual.

MTA Cooperative Group. (1999). Moderators and mediators of treatment response for children with attention-deficit/hyperactivity disorder (ADHD). *Archives of General Psychiatry, 56*(12), 1088–1096.

Robin, A. L., & Foster, S. L. (1995). The Conflict Behavior Questionnaire. In M. Hersen & A. S. Bellack (Eds.), *Dictionary of behavorial techniques* (pp. 148–150). New York: Pergamon Press.

Shaw, P., Lerch, J., Greenstein, D., Sharp, W., Clasen, L., Evans, A., et al. (2006). Longitudinal mapping of cortical thickness and clinical outcome in children and adolescents with attention-deficit/hyperactivity disorder. *Archives of General Psychiatry, 63*(5), 540–549.

Sher, K. J., Grekin, E. R., & Williams, N. A. (2005). The development of alcohol use disorders. *Annual Review of Clinical Psychology, 1*(1), 493–523.

Sibley, M. H., Altszuler, A. R., Morrow, A., & Merrill, B. (2014). Mapping the Academic Problem Behaviors of Adolescents with ADHD. *School Psychology Quarterly, 29*, 422–437.

Sibley, M. H., Campez, M., Perez, A., Morrow, A. S., Merrill, B. M., Altszuler, A. A., et al. (2016). Parent management of organization, time management, and planning deficits among adolescents with ADHD. *Journal of Psychopathology and Behavioral Assessment, 38*, 216–228.

Sibley, M. H., Graziano, P. A., Kuriyan, A. B., Coxe, S., Pelham, W. E., Rodriguez, L. M., et al. (in press). Parent–teen behavior therapy + motivational interviewing for adolescents with ADHD. *Journal of Consulting and Clinical Psychology.*

Sibley, M. H., Olson, S., Morley, C., Campez, M., & Pelham, W. E. (in press). A school consultation intervention for adolescents with ADHD: Barriers and implementation strategies. *Child and Adolescent Mental Health.*

Sibley, M. H., Pelham, W. E., Derefinko, K. D., Kuriyan, A. B., Sanchez, F., & Graziano, P. A. (2013). A pilot trial of Supporting Teens' Academic Needs Daily (STAND): A parent–adolescent collaborative intervention for ADHD. *Journal of Psychopathology and Behavioral Assessment, 35*, 436–449.

Sonuga-Barke, E. J. (2002). Psychological heterogeneity in ADHD: A dual pathway model of behaviour and cognition. *Behavioural Brain Research, 130*(1), 29–36.

Steinberg, L. (2010). *Adolescence* (9th ed.). New York: McGraw-Hill.

Steinberg, L., Lamborn, S. D., Dornbusch, S. M., & Darling, N. (1992). Impact of parenting practices on adolescent achievement: Authoritative parenting, school involvement, and encouragement to succeed. *Child Development, 63*(5), 1266–1281.

Steiner, N. J., Sheldrick, R. C., Gotthelf, D., & Perrin, E. C. (2011). Computer-based attention training in the schools for children with attention deficit/hyperactivity disorder: A preliminary trial. *Clinical Pediatrics, 50*(7), 615–622.

Swanson, J., Gupta, S., Guinta, D., Flynn, D., Agler, D., Lerner, M., et al. (1999). Acute tolerance to methylphenidate in the treatment of attention–deficit/hyperactivity disorder in children. *Clinical Pharmacology and Therapeutics, 66*(3), 295–305.

Wagner, C. C., & Ingersoll, K. S. (with Contributors). (2013). *Motivational interviewing in groups.* New York: Guilford Press.

Zucker, R. A. (2006). The developmental behavior genetics of drug involvement: Overview and comments. *Behavioral Genetics, 36*, 616–625.

Index

Page numbers followed by *f* indicate figure, *t* indicate table

Academic functioning
  adolescent period of development
    and, 5–6, 7–8, 7*f*
  case conceptualization and,
    34–35, 36*t*
  Engagement Module 1:
    Understanding the Family, 76
  interference from, 230–231
  Mobilizing Module 2: Habit
    Formation, 188–192, 190*f*
  parenting and, 11–12
  Skill Module 6: Note Taking,
    151–155, 154*f*, 155*f*
  See also Homework completion;
    Note-taking skills; Schools
Acceptance
  Engagement Module 1:
    Understanding the Family, 69
  motivational interviewing and,
    53, 54*t*, 65*t*
Accountability, 12
Action plans
  examples of, 198*f*
  Mobilizing Module 3: Making an
    Action Plan, 180*f*, 193–199,
    197, 198*f*, 199*f*
  Mobilizing Module 4: Keeping
    Momentum, 200–201
  mobilizing modules of STAND
    and, 21*t*
  overview, 197
  priority areas for, 195
  worksheets regarding, 213–215
Activities
  Engagement Module 4: Creating
    Structure at Home, 99*f*
  Skill Module 2: Making a
    Homework Plan, 135

  troubleshooting, 226–227, 228*t*
  worksheets regarding, 117
ADHD Symptom Checklist, 36*t*
Adolescent Academic Problems
  Checklist (AAPC), 35, 36*t*,
  47–48
Adolescent period of development,
  5–9, 7*f*, 9*f*, 183
Adult maladjustment, 7–8, 7*f*
Advice
  Mobilizing Module 4: Keeping
    Momentum, 204–205
  skill modules of STAND and, 128
Affirmations
  addressing disengagement and,
    218
  Mobilizing Module 2: Habit
    Formation, 188
  Mobilizing Module 4: Keeping
    Momentum, 200
  motivational interviewing and,
    65*t*, 66*t*
  overview, 56, 59, 61, 61*t*
  parental interference, 225
  skill modules of STAND and, 124
  See also Motivational
    interviewing (MI)
Ambivalence
  motivational interviewing and,
    55–56, 56*t*, 57*t*
  parental interference, 224–225
  reflections and, 62
  skill modules of STAND and,
    126*f*
Anger, 221
Anxiety, 26–27
Asking permission, 56, 58. *See also*
  Motivational interviewing (MI)

Assessment
  case conceptualization and,
    33–37, 36*t*, 37*f*, 47–50
  Engagement Module 1:
    Understanding the Family,
    69, 73
  forms for, 47–50
  measures that can be used for,
    35–37, 36*t*, 37*f*
  motivational interviewing and,
    65*t*
  Supporting Teens' Autonomy
    Daily (STAND) treatment
    model and, 21
Assignment completion. *See*
  Homework completion
Attention
  adolescent period of development
    and, 5–8
  case conceptualization and, 34, 36*t*
  classroom behavior and, 152
  comorbidities and, 26–28
  Engagement Module 1:
    Understanding the Family,
    74–75
  goals of adolescence and, 8–9
  habit formation and, 189
  homework completion and, 130,
    132
  integrated approach to
    interventions and, 18–19
  motivational interviewing and, 64
  organization skills and, 137
  overview, 4
  parental interference, 223–226
  parenting and, 11–13
  planning and decision making
    and, 156

Attention (cont.)
  time management skills and, 142
  treatment and, 9–10, 13–17, 15f, 17f
  See also Selective attention
Attention-deficit/hyperactivity
  disorder (ADHD), 15
Authoritative parenting, 11. See
  also Parenting and parenting
  patterns
Autism spectrum disorder (ASD),
  15–17
Autonomy
  adolescent period of development
    and, 5–6
  Engagement Module 2: Focusing
    Treatment Goals, 81, 87
  Mobilizing Module 1: Engaging
    the School, 181
  Mobilizing Module 2: Habit
    Formation, 188
  Mobilizing Module 4: Keeping
    Momentum, 200
  motivational interviewing and,
    65t, 66t
  parental interference, 225–226
  parenting and, 11
  session management and, 220

Backpack organization, 136–140,
  141f. See also Organizational
  skills
Behavior and behavioral problems
  addressing disengagement, 217–219
  case conceptualization and,
    34–35, 36t
  Engagement Module 1:
    Understanding the Family, 69
  overview, 4
  parenting and, 11
  Skill Module 6: Note Taking,
    151–155, 154f, 155f
  skill modules of STAND and,
    120–121
  Supporting Teens' Autonomy
    Daily (STAND) treatment
    model and, 27–28
Beliefs, 42–43
Benefits to behavior, 13–14, 15, 15f.
  See also Motivation
Blame, 218–219
Booster sessions, 29
Brain functioning, 3–5, 8–9. See also
  Neurocognitive processes
Bribery, 100

Caregiver Strain Questionnaire, 36t
Case conceptualization
  assessment and, 33–37, 36t, 37f,
    47–50
  case impression and, 37–39, 38f
  change cards and, 39, 42–44, 42f,
    43f, 44f
  Engagement Module 1:
    Understanding the Family,
    68–80, 68f, 80f
  Engagement Module 2: Focusing
    Treatment Goals, 83–84

examples of, 40f–41f
finalizing, 39, 40f–41f
motivational interviewing and, 65t
overview, 33
summarizing, 79
using to focus treatment, 45–46,
  45f
Case impression, 37–39, 38f
Change
  ambivalence and, 55–56, 56t, 57t
  Engagement Module 1:
    Understanding the Family,
    69, 77
  maintaining, 180f, 199–206,
    206f, 216
  Mobilizing Module 4: Keeping
    Momentum, 200, 201–202
  motivational interviewing and,
    65t
  readiness ruler and, 63
  See also Change cards; Change talk
Change cards
  Engagement Module 2: Focusing
    Treatment Goals, 80–89, 83f
  motivational interviewing and,
    65t
  overview, 39, 42–44, 42f, 43f, 44f
  using to focus treatment, 45
  See also Change
Change talk
  ambivalence and, 55–56, 56t, 57t
  Engagement Module 1:
    Understanding the Family, 77
  Engagement Module 2: Focusing
    Treatment Goals, 81, 84–85
  Engagement Module 3:
    Partnership Skills, 89
  Mobilizing Module 1: Engaging
    the School, 181, 184
  Mobilizing Module 2: Habit
    Formation, 188
  Mobilizing Module 4: Keeping
    Momentum, 200–201
  motivational interviewing and,
    65t, 66t
  open-ended questions to elicit, 60f
  reflecting, 61–62, 62t
  skill modules of STAND and,
    120–121, 120f, 124, 126f
Cheerleading statements, 61, 61t
Choice
  Engagement Module 2: Focusing
    Treatment Goals, 87
  Mobilizing Module 3: Making an
    Action Plan, 193
  motivational interviewing and,
    65t, 66t
  skill modules of STAND and,
    120–121
Cognitive functioning, 35–36
Cognitive training programs, 8
Collaboration
  Engagement Module 1:
    Understanding the Family, 69,
    69–72
  Engagement Module 2: Focusing
    Treatment Goals, 85

motivational interviewing and,
  65t
  See also Collaborative approach
    in STAND
Collaborative approach in parenting,
  12. See also Parenting and
  parenting patterns
Collaborative approach in STAND
  case impression and, 37–39, 38f
  Engagement Module 1:
    Understanding the Family, 69
  engagement modules of STAND
    and, 67–68
  See also Collaboration
Communication
  Engagement Module 4: Creating
    Structure at Home, 99
  engagement modules of STAND
    and, 67–68
  treatment and, 3
  worksheets regarding, 115–116
  See also "I" statements; Listening
Community-based parent training
  model, 30
Comorbidities, 26–28, 229–230
Compassion
  Engagement Module 1:
    Understanding the Family, 69
  motivational interviewing and,
    53, 54t, 55, 65t
Compensatory skills
  engagement modules of STAND
    and, 67
  goals of adolescence and, 9f
  homework completion and, 130
  interventions to help with, 10
  skill modules of STAND and,
    126f
  treatment and, 15f
Conflict Behavior Questionnaire,
  36t
Conflict during sessions, 222–223
Contingencies, 10, 14, 15f
Contracts between the parents
  and teens. See Parent–teen
  contract
Control-oriented parenting, 12–13.
  See also Parenting and
  parenting patterns

Delay aversion, 4, 13–14. See also
  Motivation
Depression, 27
Developmental processes, 5–9, 7f,
  8–9, 9f, 183
Developmental risk models, 7f
Difficulties
  Engagement Module 1:
    Understanding the Family,
    74–76
  worksheets regarding, 105
Direct observation, 34–35
Disengagement, 217–219
Disorganization. See Organizational
  skills
Displacement of blame, 218–219
Dopamine system, 6

Double-sided reflections
    motivational interviewing and, 66t
    overview, 62
    skill modules of STAND and,
        120–121
    See also Reflections

Educational accommodations, 230
Educational functioning. See
    Academic functioning
Effort, 4, 69
Elaboration
    Mobilizing Module 1: Engaging
        the School, 181
    Mobilizing Module 3: Making an
        Action Plan, 193
    motivational interviewing and,
        66t
Elicit–provide–elicit approach (EPE)
    case impression and, 38
    Engagement Module 1:
        Understanding the Family, 69,
        70, 73, 74, 76
    Engagement Module 2: Focusing
        Treatment Goals, 81, 86
    Engagement Module 3:
        Partnership Skills, 89, 91, 93
    Engagement Module 4: Creating
        Structure at Home, 97,
        100–101, 101
    Mobilizing Module 1: Engaging
        the School, 181, 184
    Mobilizing Module 2: Habit
        Formation, 188, 189–190,
        191–192
    Mobilizing Module 3: Making an
        Action Plan, 193, 196
    Mobilizing Module 4: Keeping
        Momentum, 203
    motivational interviewing and, 65t
    overview, 56, 58–59
    skill modules of STAND and,
        120–121, 120f, 125–128, 126f,
        130, 133, 137
    See also Motivational
        interviewing (MI)
Empathy
    Engagement Module 1:
        Understanding the Family, 69
    motivational interviewing and,
        65t, 66t
    parental interference, 225
    skill modules of STAND and,
        120–121
Engagement modules of STAND
    case conceptualization and, 45
    case impression and, 38–39
    change cards and, 42
    Engagement Module 1:
        Understanding the Family,
        68–80, 68f, 80f, 104–108
    Engagement Module 2: Focusing
        Treatment Goals, 68f, 80–89,
        83f, 88f, 110–113
    Engagement Module 3:
        Partnership Skills, 68f, 89–97,
        92f, 93f, 95f, 96f, 114–116, 222

Engagement Module 4: Creating
    Structure at Home, 68f,
    97–103, 99f, 103f, 117–118
    handouts and worksheets for,
        104–118
    motivational interviewing and,
        53, 57f, 64, 65t
    overview, 20f, 21–22, 67–68, 68f
    See also Supporting Teens'
        Autonomy Daily (STAND)
        treatment model
Engaging process of MI, 56, 57f. See
    also Motivational interviewing
    (MI)
Environments
    case conceptualization and, 34
    Engagement Module 4: Creating
        Structure at Home, 68f
    goals of adolescence and, 9f
    reward values and, 13–14
    Skill Module 2: Making a
        Homework Plan, 132–136,
        136f
    treatment and, 15f
    See also Home environment;
        Schools
Evocation, 54t, 55
Evoking process of MI, 56, 57f,
    97. See also Motivational
    interviewing (MI)
Executive functioning (EF)
    adolescent period of development
        and, 5–9
    case conceptualization and, 34,
        36t
    classroom behavior and, 152
    comorbidities and, 26–28
    Engagement Module 1:
        Understanding the Family,
        74–75
    habit formation and, 189
    homework completion and, 130,
        132, 133
    integrated approach to
        interventions and, 18–19
    motivational interviewing and,
        64
    organization skills and, 137
    overview, 4
    parental interference, 223–226
    parenting and, 11–13
    planning and decision making
        and, 156
    time management skills and, 142
    treatment and, 9–10, 13–17, 15f,
        17f
Expectations, 69, 228t

Family functioning
    adolescent period of development
        and, 7–8, 7f
    case impression and, 38–39
    displacement of blame and,
        218–219
    Engagement Module 1:
        Understanding the Family,
        68–80, 68f, 80f

Engagement Module 4: Creating
    Structure at Home, 68f
    engagement modules of STAND
        and, 20t
    family feedback, 79
    motivational interviewing and,
        65t, 66t
    parental interference, 223–226
    Supporting Teens' Autonomy
        Daily (STAND) treatment
        model and, 22
    troubleshooting, 226–227,
        228t–229t
Family-informed case
    conceptualization. See Case
    conceptualization
Feedback
    Engagement Module 1:
        Understanding the Family, 73,
        76, 79
    Engagement Module 3:
        Partnership Skills, 95f
    motivational interviewing and,
        65t
Flash cards
    Skill Module 5: Study Skills,
        146–151, 149f, 150f
    use of, 148
    worksheets regarding, 172–173
    See also Study skills
Focusing process of MI, 56, 57f. See
    also Motivational interviewing
    (MI)
Future goals and hopes
    Engagement Module 2: Focusing
        Treatment Goals, 80–89
    Engagement Module 3:
        Partnership Skills, 90–91
    worksheets regarding, 108–110,
        112–113
    See also Goals

Goal setting
    Engagement Module 2: Focusing
        Treatment Goals, 84–86
    goals of adolescence and, 9f
    See also Goals; Treatment goals
Goals
    Engagement Module 2: Focusing
        Treatment Goals, 68f
    goal-directed behavior, 4
    Mobilizing Module 4: Keeping
        Momentum, 202–203
    motivational interviewing and,
        52–53, 65t
    worksheets regarding, 108–110,
        112–113
    See also Future goals and hopes;
        Goal setting; Treatment goals
Grades, 35
Group format
    Engagement Module 1:
        Understanding the Family, 80f
    Engagement Module 2: Focusing
        Treatment Goals, 88f
    Engagement Module 3:
        Partnership Skills, 96f

Group format *(cont.)*
    Engagement Module 4: Creating
        Structure at Home, 103
    Mobilizing Module 1: Engaging
        the School, 187*f*
    Mobilizing Module 2: Habit
        Formation, 192*f*
    Mobilizing Module 3: Making an
        Action Plan, 199
    Mobilizing Module 4: Keeping
        Momentum, 206*f*
    Skill Module 1: Writing Down
        Homework, 132*f*
    Skill Module 2: Making a
        Homework Plan, 136*f*
    Skill Module 3: Organization
        Checkups, 141*f*
    Skill Module 4: Time
        Management Strategies, 145*f*
    Skill Module 5: Study Skills, 150*f*
    Skill Module 6: Note Taking, 155*f*
    Supporting Teens' Autonomy
        Daily (STAND) treatment
        model, 29–30, 31*t*–32*t*

Habit development
    interventions to help with, 10
    maintaining habits, 204
    Mobilizing Module 2: Habit
        Formation, 180*f*, 187–192,
        190*f*, 192*f*, 227
    Mobilizing Module 4: Keeping
        Momentum, 200–201,
        203–204
    mobilizing modules of STAND
        and, 21*t*
    worksheets regarding, 211–212
Home environment
    Engagement Module 3:
        Partnership Skills, 90–91
    Engagement Module 4: Creating
        Structure at Home, 68*f*,
        97–103, 99*f*, 103*f*
    Mobilizing Module 2: Habit
        Formation, 191–192
    mobilizing modules of STAND
        and, 180–181
    parental interference, 223–226
    troubleshooting, 226–227,
        228*t*–229*t*
    worksheets regarding, 117
    See also Environments; Structure
Home exercises
    Engagement Module 1:
        Understanding the Family, 69,
        70, 80
    Engagement Module 2: Focusing
        Treatment Goals, 89
    Engagement Module 3:
        Partnership Skills, 89, 96–97
    Engagement Module 4: Creating
        Structure at Home, 98–99, 103
    follow-through with, 122, 140
    Mobilizing Module 1: Engaging
        the School, 187
    Mobilizing Module 2: Habit
        Formation, 192

Mobilizing Module 3: Making an
        Action Plan, 199
    noncompliance with, 219
    reviewing, 121, 122–125
    Skill Module 3: Organization
        Checkups, 140
    skill modules of STAND and,
        120*f*
    troubleshooting, 227, 228*t*–229*t*
    See also Weekly skill experiments
Homework completion
    contracts and, 134–136
    Engagement Module 1:
        Understanding the Family,
        69–72, 74–76, 77–79
    Engagement Module 2: Focusing
        Treatment Goals, 83–84, 86
    Engagement Module 4: Creating
        Structure at Home, 97–103,
        99*f*, 103*f*
    homework plan, 20*t*
    Mobilizing Module 2: Habit
        Formation, 188–192, 190*f*
    Skill Module 1: Writing Down
        Homework, 129–132, 132*f*
    Skill Module 2: Making a
        Homework Plan, 132–136,
        136*f*
    Skill Module 4: Time
        Management Strategies,
        141–145, 145*f*
    skill modules of STAND and, 20*t*
    treatment and, 3
    worksheets regarding, 160–163
    See also Academic functioning
Hope, 80–89, 108–110, 112–113

"I" statements
    Engagement Module 3:
        Partnership Skills, 89, 94–96,
        95*f*
    worksheets regarding, 115
    See also Communication
Identity formation, 9*f*
Impulse control, 6–7
Independence
    adolescent period of development
        and, 5–7
    Engagement Module 2: Focusing
        Treatment Goals, 84
    Engagement Module 4: Creating
        Structure at Home, 101
    goals of adolescence and, 9, 9*f*
    interventions to help with, 10
    Mobilizing Module 1: Engaging
        the School, 183
Individualization, 19–20
Integrated approach, 18–19. *See also*
        Treatment
Interests
    case conceptualization and, 34
    interventions to help with, 10
Interfering factors, 229–231
Interparental discord, 223
Interventions, 9–10, 14. *See also*
        Treatment modalities
Interviews, 35, 36*t*, 37*f*

Life events, 9*f*, 10. *See also* Stress
Limit setting
    Engagement Module 3:
        Partnership Skills, 90–91
    parental fear of, 224–225
    parenting and, 12
Limit testing, 9*f*
Listening
    Engagement Module 1:
        Understanding the Family, 69
    Engagement Module 3:
        Partnership Skills, 89, 93–94,
        93*f*
    motivational interviewing and,
        65*t*, 66*t*
    worksheets regarding, 115
    See also Communication

Materials needed to conduct STAND
    Engagement Module 1:
        Understanding the Family, 68
    Engagement Module 2: Focusing
        Treatment Goals, 80
    Engagement Module 3:
        Partnership Skills, 89
    Engagement Module 4: Creating
        Structure at Home, 97
    Mobilizing Module 1: Engaging
        the School, 181
    Mobilizing Module 2: Habit
        Formation, 187
    Mobilizing Module 3: Making an
        Action Plan, 193
    Mobilizing Module 4: Keeping
        Momentum, 199
    overview, 22–23
    Skill Module 1: Writing Down
        Homework, 129
    Skill Module 2: Making a
        Homework Plan, 132
    Skill Module 3: Organization
        Checkups, 136
    Skill Module 4: Time
        Management Strategies, 141
    Skill Module 5: Study Skills, 146
    Skill Module 6: Note Taking, 151
    Skill Module 7: Problem Solving,
        155
    See also Worksheets
Medications, 8
Mobilizing change talk
    Engagement Module 2: Focusing
        Treatment Goals, 81
    Mobilizing Module 1: Engaging
        the School, 181
    Mobilizing Module 4: Keeping
        Momentum, 200–201
    open-ended questions to elicit, 60*f*
    skill modules of STAND and,
        120–121, 124
    See also Change talk
Mobilizing modules of STAND
    handouts and worksheets for,
        207–216
    Mobilizing Module 1: Engaging
        the School, 180*f*, 181–187,
        185*f*, 187*f*, 207–210

Mobilizing Module 2: Habit Formation, 180*f*, 187–192, 190*f*, 192*f*, 211–212, 227
Mobilizing Module 3: Making an Action Plan, 180*f*, 193–199, 198*f*, 199*f*, 213–215
Mobilizing Module 4: Keeping Momentum, 180*f*, 199–206, 206*f*, 216
motivational interviewing and, 53, 57*f*, 64, 66*t*
overview, 21*f*, 22, 180–181, 180*f*
See also Supporting Teens' Autonomy Daily (STAND) treatment model
Momentum
Mobilizing Module 4: Keeping Momentum, 180*f*, 199–206, 206*f*
worksheets regarding, 216
Motivation
adolescent period of development and, 5–8
case conceptualization and, 34, 36*t*
classroom behavior and, 152
comorbidities and, 26–28
Engagement Module 1: Understanding the Family, 74–75
engagement modules of STAND and, 67
goals of adolescence and, 8–9
habit formation and, 189
homework completion and, 130, 132
integrated approach to interventions and, 18–19
organization skills and, 137
overview, 4, 13–14
parental interference, 223–226
parenting and, 11–13
planning and decision making and, 156
time management skills and, 142
treatment and, 9–10, 13–17, 15*f*, 17*f*
See also Delay aversion
Motivational interviewing (MI)
ambivalence and, 55–56, 56*t*, 57*t*
core MI skills, 56, 58–64, 60*f*, 61*t*, 62*t*
Engagement Module 1: Understanding the Family, 69, 70
Engagement Module 3: Partnership Skills, 89
Engagement Module 4: Creating Structure at Home, 97
motivational interviewing and, 64
overview, 14
process goals of, 56, 57*f*
in STAND, 52–55, 54*t*, 64–65, 65*t*–66*t*
Supporting Teens' Autonomy Daily (STAND) treatment model and, 23

training and integrity in implementation of, 64–65
treatment and, 15*f*
Motivational Interviewing Network of Trainers (MINT), 64–65
Multicomponent approach, 18–19. *See also* Treatment
Multimodal Treatment Study of Children with ADHD (MTA study), 8

Negative parent–child cycles, 11–13. *See also* Parenting and parenting patterns
Neurocognitive processes
adolescent period of development and, 5–6, 8–9, 9*f*
interventions to help with, 10
overview, 3–5
See also Brain functioning
Nonparticipation, 217–219
Note-taking skills
benefits of note taking and, 152
overview, 154*f*
Skill Module 5: Study Skills, 148–149, 149*f*
Skill Module 6: Note Taking, 151–155, 154*f*, 155*f*
skill modules of STAND and, 20*t*
worksheets regarding, 174, 176–177
See also Academic functioning

Observation, 34–35, 36*t*
Open-ended questions
addressing disengagement and, 217
Engagement Module 2: Focusing Treatment Goals, 84–85
Mobilizing Module 1: Engaging the School, 184
overview, 56, 59, 60*f*, 66*t*
summaries and, 63
See also Motivational interviewing (MI)
Oppositional behavior, 27–28
Organization checkup, 136–140, 141*f*
Organizational skills
adolescent period of development and, 6
Engagement Module 1: Understanding the Family, 69–72
interventions to help with, 10
parenting and, 12
of parents, 223–224
Skill Module 3: Organization Checkups, 136–140, 141*f*
skill modules of STAND and, 20*t*
Supporting Teens' Autonomy Daily (STAND) treatment model and, 16–17, 17*f*
treatment and, 3
worksheets regarding, 164–167

Parent Academic Management Scale (PAMS), 35, 36*t*, 49–50
Parental control pattern of parenting, 12–13. *See also* Parenting and parenting patterns
Parenting and parenting patterns
Engagement Module 1: Understanding the Family, 69, 76–79
motivational interviewing and, 65*t*
overview, 11–13
parental interference, 223–226
perceived reward values and, 14
Supporting Teens' Autonomy Daily (STAND) treatment model and, 16–17, 21
treatment and, 15*f*
troubleshooting, 226–227, 228*t*–229*t*
worksheets regarding, 106–107
Parents
ambivalence and, 55–56, 56*t*, 57*t*
case conceptualization and, 34, 36*t*
case impression and, 37–39, 38*f*
change cards and, 42–43, 44, 82
conflict between, 223
displacement of blame and, 218–219
Engagement Module 1: Understanding the Family, 68–80, 68*f*, 69, 72–74, 80*f*
Engagement Module 2: Focusing Treatment Goals, 81, 82, 84–85
engagement modules of STAND and, 67–68
involvement in STAND, 25
mental health of, 3
motivational interviewing and, 52–53, 65*t*
parental interference, 223–226
reflecting change talk and, 61–62, 62*t*
session management, 219–223
Skill Module 2: Making a Homework Plan, 132–136, 136*f*
skill modules of STAND and, 120*f*
as stakeholders, 11
See also Parenting and parenting patterns; Parent–teen relationship
Parent–teen contract
Engagement Module 4: Creating Structure at Home, 97–103, 99*f*, 103*f*
Mobilizing Module 2: Habit Formation, 192
practice plans as, 119
refusal to sign, 219–221
Skill Module 1: Writing Down Homework, 130–131
Skill Module 2: Making a Homework Plan, 134–136
worksheets regarding, 118, 161, 163, 167, 170, 177, 179
See also Parent–teen partnership

Parent–teen meeting
    Engagement Module 3:
        Partnership Skills, 89, 96–97
    Engagement Module 4: Creating
        Structure at Home, 98–99
    worksheets regarding, 116
Parent–teen partnership
    Engagement Module 3:
        Partnership Skills, 68f, 89–97,
        91, 92f, 93f, 95f, 96f
    engagement modules of STAND
        and, 67–68
    motivational interviewing and,
        65t
    See also Parent–teen contract;
        Parent–teen relationship;
        Partnership
Parent–teen relationship
    case conceptualization and, 36t
    conflict during sessions and,
        222
    Engagement Module 3:
        Partnership Skills, 91–93, 92f
    motivational interviewing and,
        52–53
    overview, 11
    parenting patterns and, 13
    Supporting Teens' Autonomy
        Daily (STAND) treatment
        model and, 22
    treatment and, 3
    See also Parents; Parent–teen
        partnership
Partnership
    Engagement Module 1:
        Understanding the Family,
        69–72
    Engagement Module 3:
        Partnership Skills, 68f, 89–97,
        92f, 93f, 95f, 96f, 222
    engagement modules of STAND
        and, 20t
    motivational interviewing and,
        53, 54t, 65t
    overview, 21
    See also Parent–teen partnership
Pay-offs. See Perceived reward values
Peer relationships, 7–8, 7f, 34
Perceived reward values, 13–14, 15,
    15f. See also Motivation
Permission, asking. See Asking
    permission
Personal assistant parenting,
    12–13. See also Parenting and
    parenting patterns
Persuasion, 128
Philosophical differences, 224
Planner use
    Skill Module 1: Writing Down
        Homework, 129–132, 132f
    Skill Module 4: Time
        Management Strategies,
        141–145, 145f
    See also Planning skills
Planning process of MI, 56, 57f. See
    also Motivational interviewing
    (MI)

Planning skills
    adolescent period of development
        and, 6
    interventions to help with, 10
    parenting and, 12
    Skill Module 7: Problem Solving,
        155–159, 157f, 158f
    Supporting Teens' Autonomy
        Daily (STAND) treatment
        model and, 16–17, 17f
    treatment and, 3
    See also Planner use
Point person, 184–185
Positive changes. See Change
Practice
    interventions to help with, 10
    Mobilizing Module 4: Keeping
        Momentum, 203–204
    reinforcing, 13
    skill modules of STAND and,
        119
    See also Practice plan; Skill
        practice
Practice monitoring, 196
Practice plan
    Skill Module 1: Writing Down
        Homework, 130–131
    Skill Module 2: Making a
        Homework Plan, 133–134
    Skill Module 3: Organization
        Checkups, 138–140
    Skill Module 4: Time
        Management Strategies,
        143–144
    Skill Module 5: Study Skills,
        147–149, 149f
    Skill Module 6: Note Taking, 153
    Skill Module 7: Problem Solving,
        157, 157f, 158f
    skill modules of STAND and, 119,
        120f, 128
    worksheets regarding, 160, 162,
        165–166
    See also Practice
Preparatory change talk, 60f, 81. See
    also Change talk
Pretreatment interview, 35
Priorities
    action plans and, 195
    Engagement Module 1:
        Understanding the Family, 69
    motivational interviewing and,
        65t
Problem solving skills
    overview, 157f, 158f
    Skill Module 7: Problem Solving,
        155–159, 157f, 158f
    skill modules of STAND and,
        20t
    worksheets regarding, 178–179
Procrastination, 3
Pseudo-word activity, 147, 173
Psychosocial history, 36t

Questions, open-ended. See Open-
    ended questions
Quick Delay Questionnaire, 36t

Readiness ruler
    Engagement Module 2: Focusing
        Treatment Goals, 81, 84–85
    overview, 56, 63, 66t
    skill modules of STAND and, 120
    See also Motivational
        interviewing (MI)
Reading notes
    Skill Module 5: Study Skills,
        148–149, 149f
    worksheets regarding, 174
    See also Note-taking skills
Record review, 36t
Reflections
    Engagement Module 1:
        Understanding the Family, 69
    Engagement Module 2: Focusing
        Treatment Goals, 81
    Mobilizing Module 1: Engaging
        the School, 184
    Mobilizing Module 4: Keeping
        Momentum, 200–201
    motivational interviewing and,
        65t, 66t
    overview, 56, 61–62, 62t
    session management and, 222
    skill modules of STAND and,
        120–121
    summaries and, 63
    See also Motivational
        interviewing (MI)
Reflective listening
    Engagement Module 3:
        Partnership Skills, 89, 93–94,
        93f
    worksheets regarding, 115
    See also Listening
Reframing
    change cards and, 42–43
    motivational interviewing and,
        66t
Reinforcement
    skill modules of STAND and, 120f
    troubleshooting, 228t
Relationships, 5. See also Parent–
    teen relationship; Peer
    relationships
Reluctance, 217–219
Responsibilities
    displacement of blame and,
        218–219
    Engagement Module 4: Creating
        Structure at Home, 97–103,
        99f, 103f
    skill modules of STAND and, 129
    worksheets regarding, 117
Restrictions, 229t
Reviewing lessons, 66t, 121, 122–125
Rewards, 100, 225. See also
    Perceived reward values
Routines
    Mobilizing Module 2: Habit
        Formation, 187–192, 190f,
        191–192, 192f
    Mobilizing Module 3: Making an
        Action Plan, 193–199, 198f,
        199f

Mobilizing Module 4: Keeping
   Momentum, 200
mobilizing modules of STAND
   and, 180–181
motivational interviewing and,
   66t
parents participating in STAND
   and, 25
remembering to bring materials to
   sessions and, 23
Skill Module 2: Making a
   Homework Plan, 132–136,
   136f
Skill Module 4: Time
   Management Strategies,
   141–145, 145f
treatment and, 3
See also Home environment;
   Schools; Structure

Scaling questions, 86
School staff, 181–187, 185f, 187f
Schools
   adolescent period of development
      and, 6, 7–8, 7f
   case conceptualization and,
      34–35
   interference from, 230–231
   Mobilizing Module 1: Engaging
      the School, 180f, 181–187,
      185f, 187f
   Mobilizing Module 2: Habit
      Formation, 188–192, 190f
   mobilizing modules of STAND
      and, 21t
   overview, 183
   Supporting Teens' Autonomy
      Daily (STAND) treatment
      model and, 22
   worksheets regarding, 207–210
   See also Academic functioning;
      Environments
Selective attention, 4. See also
   Attention
Self-efficacy, 14, 15f
Self-evaluation, 65
Self-management skills, 6
Self-regulation, 7–8, 11
Self-sufficiency, 9f, 196
Session management, 219–223
Skill development, 9f
Skill modules of STAND
   Engagement Module 2: Focusing
      Treatment Goals, 80–89,
      86–89, 88f
   Mobilizing Module 2: Habit
      Formation, 190–191, 190f
   motivational interviewing and,
      57f, 64, 65t, 66t
   overview, 20f, 22, 119–129, 121f,
      126f
   Skill Module 1: Writing Down
      Homework, 120f, 129–132,
      132f, 160–161
   Skill Module 2: Making a
      Homework Plan, 120f,
      132–136, 136f, 162–163

Skill Module 3: Organization
   Checkups, 120f, 136–140, 141f,
   164–167
Skill Module 4: Time
   Management Strategies, 120f,
   141–145, 145f, 168–170
Skill Module 5: Study Skills, 120f,
   146–151, 149f, 150f, 171–175
Skill Module 6: Note Taking,
   120f, 151–155, 154f, 155f,
   176–177
Skill Module 7: Problem Solving,
   120f, 155–159, 157f, 158f,
   178–179
worksheets regarding, 111,
   160–179
See also Supporting Teens'
   Autonomy Daily (STAND)
   treatment model
Skill practice
   Mobilizing Module 2: Habit
      Formation, 190–191, 190f
   Mobilizing Module 4: Keeping
      Momentum, 203–204
   motivational interviewing and,
      66t
   noncompliance with, 219
   open-ended questions and, 60f
   skill instruction and, 10, 13, 66t
   skill modules of STAND and, 120f
   troubleshooting, 229t
   See also Practice; Skill use
Skill use
   motivational interviewing and,
      66t
   open-ended questions and, 60f
   troubleshooting, 228t
   See also Skill practice
Skills-based treatment, 64
Social functioning, 5–6, 7–8, 7f
STAND treatment model. See
   Supporting Teens' Autonomy
   Daily (STAND) treatment
   model
Stimulant medications, 8
Strengths
   adolescent period of development
      and, 5
   case conceptualization and, 34,
      36t
   Engagement Module 1: Under-
      standing the Family, 69, 72–74
   goals of adolescence and, 9
   motivational interviewing and, 65t
   worksheets regarding, 105
Stress
   case conceptualization and, 36t
   Engagement Module 3: Partner-
      ship Skills, 89, 91–93, 92f
   treatment and, 3
   worksheets regarding, 114
Structure
   Engagement Module 3:
      Partnership Skills, 90–91
   Engagement Module 4: Creating
      Structure at Home, 68f,
      97–103, 99f, 103f

engagement modules of STAND
   and, 20t
mobilizing modules of STAND
   and, 180–181
parental interference, 223–226
parenting and, 12
removing too early, 227
treatment and, 3
troubleshooting, 226–227,
   228t–229t
worksheets regarding, 117
See also Home environment;
   Routines
Study skills
   Engagement Module 2: Focusing
      Treatment Goals, 86
   Skill Module 5: Study Skills,
      146–151, 149f, 150f
   skill modules of STAND and,
      20t
   worksheets regarding, 171–175
Summaries, 56, 63–64, 69, 79. See
   also Motivational interviewing
   (MI)
Supporting Teens' Autonomy Daily
   (STAND) treatment model
   addressing disengagement,
      217–219
   appropriate ages for, 24–25
   booster sessions and, 29
   case conceptualization and, 33,
      45–46, 45f
   comorbidities and, 26–28
   delivery of, 23
   empirical support for, 16–17, 17f
   in a group format, 29–30, 31t–32t
   materials for, 22–23
   motivational interviewing and,
      52–55, 54t, 56, 57f, 64–65,
      65t–66t
   outcomes, 28
   overview, 15–17, 15f, 17f, 18–19,
      30
   participating parents, 25
   session structure, 19–22, 20t–21t,
      219–223
   treatment goals and, 26
   See also Engagement modules of
      STAND; Mobilizing modules
      of STAND; Skill modules of
      STAND

Teachers
   case conceptualization and,
      34–35, 36t
   Mobilizing Module 1: Engaging
      the School, 181–187, 185f, 187f
   Mobilizing Module 2: Habit
      Formation, 188–192, 190f
   Skill Module 1: Writing Down
      Homework, 131
Teens
   addressing disengagement and,
      217–219
   ambivalence and, 55–56, 56t, 57t
   case conceptualization and, 36t
   change cards and, 44

Teens *(cont.)*
    displacement of blame and,
        218–219
    Engagement Module 1:
        Understanding the Family,
        72–74
    Engagement Module 2: Focusing
        Treatment Goals, 81, 84–85
    Mobilizing Module 1: Engaging
        the School, 183
    motivational interviewing and,
        52–53, 65*t*
    session management, 219–223
    Skill Module 2: Making a Home-
        work Plan, 132–136, 136*f*
    skill modules of STAND and, 120*f*
Termination, 206, 231
Therapist contact note, 45*f*, 46. *See
    also* Case conceptualization
Therapist's role, 69
Time management skills
    adolescent period of development
        and, 6
    Engagement Module 2: Focusing
        Treatment Goals, 86
    interventions to help with, 10
    parenting and, 12
    Skill Module 4: Time
        Management Strategies,
        141–145, 145*f*
    skill modules of STAND and, 20*t*
    Supporting Teens' Autonomy
        Daily (STAND) treatment
        model and, 16–17, 17*f*
    treatment and, 3
    worksheets regarding, 168–170
Toolbox of skills, 190–191, 190*f*
Treatment, 45–46, 45*f*. *See also*
    Supporting Teens' Autonomy
    Daily (STAND) treatment
    model
Treatment goals
    Engagement Module 2: Focusing
        Treatment Goals, 68*f*, 80–89
    engagement modules of STAND
        and, 20*t*

motivational interviewing and,
    65*t*
Supporting Teens' Autonomy
    Daily (STAND) treatment
    model and, 26
See also Goals
Treatment menu, 65*t*. *See also* Skill
    modules of STAND; Skill
    practice
Treatment modalities
    engaging parents in, 11
    goals of adolescence and, 8
    overview, 3, 9–10, 15–17, 15*f*, 17*f*
    See also Interventions
Treatment planning, 21. *See also*
    Case conceptualization

Understanding, 65*t*, 69
Uninvolved parenting, 12–13. *See
    also* Parenting and parenting
    patterns

Values
    case conceptualization and, 34,
        36*t*
    change cards and, 42–43
    Engagement Module 1:
        Understanding the Family, 69
    interventions to help with, 10
    motivational interviewing and,
        65*t*
    worksheets regarding, 104
Visual aids, 73

Weekly skill experiments
    motivational interviewing and,
        66*t*
    open-ended questions and, 60*f*
    overview, 129
    Skill Module 2: Making a
        Homework Plan, 134–136
    Skill Module 3: Organization
        Checkups, 137, 140
    Skill Module 4: Time
        Management Strategies, 145
    Skill Module 5: Study Skills, 146

Skill Module 6: Note Taking, 151,
    153–155, 154*f*
Skill Module 7: Problem Solving,
    156, 159
See also Home exercises; Skill
    practice
Worksheets
    Adolescent Academic Problems
        Checklist (AAPC), 47–48
    Engagement Module 1:
        Understanding the Family, 68,
        104–109
    Engagement Module 2: Focusing
        Treatment Goals, 80, 110–113
    Engagement Module 3:
        Partnership Skills, 89, 114–116
    Engagement Module 4: Creating
        Structure at Home, 97, 117–118
    Mobilizing Module 1: Engaging
        the School, 181, 207–210
    Mobilizing Module 2: Habit
        Formation, 187, 211–212
    Mobilizing Module 3: Making an
        Action Plan, 193, 213–215
    Mobilizing Module 4: Keeping
        Momentum, 199, 216
    overview, 22–23
    Parent Academic Management
        Scale (PAMS), 49–50
    Skill Module 1: Writing Down
        Homework, 129, 160–161
    Skill Module 2: Making a
        Homework Plan, 132, 162–163
    Skill Module 3: Organization
        Checkups, 136, 164–167
    Skill Module 4: Time
        Management Strategies, 141,
        168–170
    Skill Module 5: Study Skills, 146,
        171–175
    Skill Module 6: Note Taking, 151,
        176–177
    Skill Module 7: Problem Solving,
        155, 178–179
    See also Materials needed to
        conduct STAND